For Sophie and Adam, thanks for everything.

Sleep is an essential life habit and is closely associated with lifespan, diabetes, hypertension, and mental health…

Plus a whole lot more

Imagine a disease so aggressive that it can have damaging effects to every single body system that we possess.

Imagine this same condition is not well recognised by health care professionals, which means it is under-diagnosed and under-treated.

Imagine this disease is so common that about 20% of children have it, and 20-40% of adults have it.

Imagine we have known about this condition for centuries.

Imagine, that the way we diagnose it is flawed and that the way it is treated is also flawed.

Imagine, that if I told you the name of this condition, that most health care providers could not explain what it was.

This is the conundrum of sleep disordered breathing, a medical condition characterised by an inability to breathe properly at the time a person is asleep. A condition that results in low levels of oxygen throughout the body. A disease that causes bodily damage that is totally avoidable.

This book should not even need to exist, but here it is. This book aims to change the way people look at snoring, mouth breathing, and obstructive sleep apnoea. All of these are part of the sleep disordered breathing spectrum.

The following pages will explore this disease in greater detail. A significant number of known medical condition related to sleep disordered breathing is defined and explained and references are provided to allow further exploration on the topic. Not every single condition is covered, which goes to show just how significant this disease process is; there is a blend of the rare and the common to give a broad narrative to the discussion. The intention is to be concise and precise.

Once you have read through this book, I believe you will agree- DON'T IGNORE THE SNORE!!

About the Author

Dr David McIntosh is a paediatric ear nose and throat (ENT) doctor in Australia. He is the go-to person for many healthcare professionals all over the world when it comes to understanding the links between nocturnal obstructed breathing and health outcomes. Apart from his clinical work, David is already the author of another book- "*Snored to Death*". In this book he describes the causes of upper airway obstruction, how to assess for it, and the treatment pathways that may be considered for resolving the disease process. This current book is an excellent complement to his first book and readers are encouraged to indulge in both this book and *Snored to Death*.

From 2021, David will also be involved in the running of a holistic health centre that will see an integration of physical exercise, mediation, breathing training, diet and nutrition and sleep health. The centre will be known as the *Synergy Performance Institute*.

Resources:

Facebook:

Snored to Death- the Book

Dr David McIntosh

Don't Ignore the Snore- the book

Synergy Performance Institute

Instagram

dr_david_mcintosh_ent

syneryperformance institute

Youtube

ENT Specialists

Synergy Performance Institute

Books

Snored to death is available from its Facebook page for a hard copy and it is also available on Amazon at https://a.co/c6Lm8Sp

Contents

1. Academic Issues...12

2. Acid Reflux 14

3. Aggressive behaviour..16

4. Alzheimer's Disease 18

5. Angina and coronary artery disease 20

6. Anxiety disorder..22

7. Aortic Aneurysm..24

8. Asthma 26

9. Atrial Fibrillation...28

10. Atrioventricular Block...30

11. Attention Deficit Hyperactivity Disorder (ADHD).........32

12. Barret's Oesophagus 34

13. Bedwetting 36

14. Benign Prostatic Hyperplasia 38

15 Bipolar Disease 40

16. Breast Cancer 42

17. Central Serous Chorioretinopathy 44

18. Cerebrovascular Disease 46

19. Chipped Teeth and bruxism 48

20. Chronic Headaches..50

21. Chronic Kidney Disease...52

22. Cognitive Impairment 54

23. Decayed Teeth..56

24. Decreased exercise tolerance....................................58

25. Decreased Libido...60

26. Dental Malocclusion 62

27. Depression...64

28. Diabetes..66

29. Difficult Pregnancy 68

30. Dry Eye Syndrome 70

31. Eczema 72

32. Elevated Cholesterol 74

33. Epilepsy...76

34. Erectile Dysfunction..78

35. Excessive Daytime Sleepiness 80

36. Fibromyalgia 82

37. Floppy Eyelid Syndrome...84

38. Glaucoma 86

39. Growth impairment 88

40. Gut Dysbiosis 90

41. Hearing Loss 92

42. High Blood Pressure...94

43. Hypercoagulable Disorder..96

44. Hypothyroidism..98

45. Irritable Bowel Syndrome 100

46. Leg Cramps at Night 102

47. Low Testosterone 104

48. Melanoma...106

49. Multiple Sclerosis..108

50. Nocturia..110

51. Non-alcoholic Fatty Liver Disease............................112

52. Non-arteritic Anterior Ischaemic Optic Neuropathy 114

53. Overactive Bladder Syndrome 116

54. Parkinson's Disease..118

55. Periodontal Disease 120

56. Polycystic Ovary Syndrome 122

57. Psychosis..124

58. Schizophrenia 126

59. Systemic Lupus Erythematosus....................................128

References 130

1. Academic Issues

In a famously titled article "On Some Causes of Backwardness and Stupidity in Children: And the Relife of these Symptoms in Some Instances by Naso-Pharyngeal Scarifications" written by William Hill in 1889, there is a similarly famously quoted passage:

"The stupid-looking lazy child who frequently suffers from headaches at school, breathes through his mouth instead of his nose, snores and is restless at night, and wakes up with a dry mouth in the morning, is well worthy of the solicitous attention of the school medical officer" (1).

Though obviously not meeting the standards of modern-day political correctness, the observation being made is pertinent- children that cannot breathe properly are likely to be struggling at school.

The Science

It is extraordinary that the observations made over 100 years ago continue to be validated by modern day research.

Scientists in Finland have recently shown that children that are simply snoring are having problems with their attention and focus during the day (2).

In New Zealand researches focussed on three elements of learning: reading, writing and math (3). Their findings were startling. In children aged between 6-10 years, the rate of learning problems with each of these was about twice the rate in children with breathing problems at night compared to normal breathing children.

Children in China were also likewise found to be struggling at school if they could not breathe properly, with the added issues of loneliness and depression also manifesting in such children (4).

A meta-analysis of the published literature brings this topic all together in their simple summary at the end:

"the findings serve to highlight to parents, teachers, and clinicians that SDB *[sleep disordered breathing]* in children may contribute to academic difficulties some children face" (5).

2. Acid Reflux

When we swallow food, it is pushed down the oesophagus and through into the stomach. Gastroesophageal reflux describes the situation where the stomach acid flows back into the oesophagus, sometimes reaching as high as the throat (and even the ears!).

Gastroesophageal reflux is considered moderate to severe acid if it occurs at least once a week. The management of gastroesophageal reflux includes lifestyle changes and medications, sometimes surgery.

The most common symptoms of gastroesophageal reflux include heartburn creating a feeling of burning rising up from the stomach to the chest, regurgitation back up the mouth causing an unpleasant bitter taste, and pain when swallowing.

As the acid reflux can get into the throat, it can also sometimes reach into the nose and across to the ears. This can cause additional symptoms such as a cough, croaky voice, feeling of a lump in the throat, nasal congestion, post-nasal drip, and blocked ears. This type of reflux is called laryngopharyngeal reflux.

The Science

There are two perspectives on the discussion on the science of acid reflux and upper airway obstruction. One is the presences of upper airway obstruction in those with reflux, and the other is the presence of reflux in those with upper airway obstruction.

To the first point, in those primarily diagnosed with upper airway obstruction, Chinese research showed that there was an elevated possibility of patients with reflux having upper airway obstruction, with the numbers being twice that in those with reflux compared to those that did not (6).

To the second point, in those primarily diagnosed with upper airway obstruction, Turkish research showed a significant rate of both gastroesophageal reflux and laryngopharyngeal reflux in the patients with obstructive sleep apnoea (7). What is interesting about this though, is that it is the more presence of upper airway obstruction, rather than the severity of the upper airway obstruction, that seems to be important (8).

Looking at the topic more broadly, meta-analysis of the published literature confirms an association between acid reflux and upper airway obstruction (9), and that the use of continuous positive airway pressure reduces the reflux symptoms (10) (11).

3. Aggressive behaviour

For anyone, adult or child, that has a single bad night's sleep, there is a good chance that person will be grumpy and moody and emotional and may well be prone to acting out in an angry fashion, running on a short fuse. It is no wonder then that if there is a chronic sleep problem, that the day time functioning level of an individual experiencing poor sleep quality will be less than optimal.

The Science

In 2007, scientists in New York estimated that in the United States alone there were 15 million children experiencing some form of poor sleep, with a particular focus on inadequate sleep being a major issue (12). Further research from the United States quantified the increased likelihood of a child having anger management issues being 40-80% more likely if they were not getting adequate sleep (13).

Chinese research has taken our understanding of the observed aggressive behaviour in children with upper airway obstruction to a whole new level, performing brain wave monitoring during sleep and noting differences in those children with airway obstruction to those without (14). They found that the frontal cortex of the brain, the area that controls behaviour, as indeed dysfunctional.

This aggressive behaviour is not a trivial issue. Research has shown that children that are identified as being trouble makers at school have a high rate of airway obstruction (15).

4. Alzheimer's Disease

Alzheimer's disease is an incurable and irreversible brain disease. There are growing numbers of cases and it represents a significant public health concern.

Alzheimer's disease slowly destroys memory and thinking skills, leading to the inability to carry out the routine tasks.

The disease starts in a part of the brain known as the hippocampus, which is the part responsible for memories. It is characterised by a build-up of lumps of protein plaques known as amyloid, and tangles of strands of protein known as neurofibrillary bundles, or tau. Another feature is the loss of connections between the brain cells.

The Science

The relationship of Alzheimer's disease to obstructive sleep apnoea is well known. Doctors from the Alzheimer's Disease Center at the NYU Langone Medical Center (16) have highlighted that obstructive sleep apnoea is associated with disruptions of sleep architecture, intermittent low oxygen levels, and oxidative stress. Researchers at the Sleep and Brain Plasticity Centre at King's College London feel this and systemic inflammation and obesity, are likely to interfere with immunological processes of the brain, and together they may promote disease progression (17).

It has also been noted that the presence of cognitive impairment affects sleep quality in its own right. The team of researchers at the Department of Psychiatry of the Harvard Medical School have noted that a decline in sleep quality contributes to a deterioration in mental function by a far greater extent when there is already pre-existing neurodegenerative disease (18). This suggests there may be a vicious circle of poor sleep, brain damage, and worse sleep.

While there has been much speculation, a ground breaking finding was that of the Alzheimer's Disease Neuroimaging Initiative (19) where they noted the presence of SDB was associated with an earlier age at which there was evidence cognitive decline. In what may be a small glimmer of hope though, for those that were treated with CPAP, their disease severity seemed to be less than those that were not being actively treated.

5. Angina and coronary artery disease

Angina is the medical term describing the chest pain experienced by patients with inadequate oxygenation of their heart muscles. It further medical terminology, this inadequate amount of oxygen is called ischeamia, and the proper term is ischaemic heart disease.

The most common reason that patients experience ischaemic heart disease is because the blood vessels that carry blood in to the heart muscle itself are blocked, either in part or in totality. If there is a complete blockage for a period of time, the muscle of the heart will die due to the lack of adequate oxygen. This is known as a heart attack, or a myocardial infarction to share the medical terminology once again.

The blood vessels to the heart will become narrow due to a build up of debris known as plaque within the blood vessel wall. There are many known risk factors for this, and it includes having high blood pressure, diabetes, high cholesterol, increasing age, a family history of the disease and being male. Many of these factors are implicated as consequence of upper airway obstruction.

The Science

Scientific research from Korea has shown that having obstructive sleep apnoea is a risk factor for the progression of sub-clinical plaque build up within the blood vessels of the heart- it is this plaque that leads to narrowing of the blood vessels and hence a reduction in blood flow to the heart muscle (20).

The importance of detecting obstructive sleep apnoea is very relevant in those that end up suffering from cardiac ischeamia and need rehabilitation from their disease (21). The Lithuanian clinicians that looked in to this found that if a patient had coronary artery disease and had undiagnosed obstructive sleep apnoea, the outcomes were worse than those having their obstructive sleep apnoea identified and managed

The corollary is also true- those with obstructive sleep apnoea need to be screened for coronary artery disease due to the high likelihood of both diseases co-existing (22)

6. Anxiety disorder

Having a state of mind that is preoccupied with worry and angst is typical of those living with anxiety disorder. Anxiety is your body's natural response to stress. It becomes a disorder if the feelings are extreme, last for more than six months, and are interfering with your daily life.

The part of the brain that is responsible for anxiety is the amygdala. In previous lifetimes, some sense of angst was appropriate in the context of such angst being related to being vigilant for predatory animals viewing us as a food source. With those sorts of threats removed from our modern way of living, the brain has found a new use for this component, turning everyday situations into potential threats that are more about perception than reality.

The Science

In patients who have trouble breathing at night, it is the equivalent as someone choking them, though of course they are their own assailant in this regard. This repeated experience leads to the brain learning to embrace worry and the anxiety then overflows in to the day.

Whilst this logical premise makes sense, it has been difficult for the science to support the notion that obstructed breathing does indeed increase the likelihood of developing an anxiety disorder (23).

A recent epidemiological study in Greece of close to 1,000 people has, however, helps bring the concept into reality (24). In their research they found anxiety was not only related to obstructive sleep apnoea but also insomnia.

Spanish researchers have taken this one step further and found that for those with moderate obstructive sleep apnoea, the use of continuous positive airway pressure therapy had a beneficial impact on reducing the level of anxiety that their test subjects were experiencing (25).

7. Aortic Aneurysm

When the blood pumps blood around, it pumps it out of the heat into blood vessels known as arteries. The major artery in the body is called the aorta. This blood vessel is connected to the left ventricle. Arteries are the strongest blood vessels in the body, a requirement of necessity as they need to absorb the force that comes from the blood being under very high pressure.

Despite their strength, arteries are vulnerable to damage and can deteriorate over time. In circumstances where they lose their integrity and strength, their diminished resilience results in their walls stretching. This in turn means the calibre of the blood vessel increases and this dilatation of the blood vessel is known as an aneurysm.

When the aorta develops an aneurysm, there is a risk that the weakness then resulted in this outcome can progress to the point that the blood vessel can rupture, causing significant and often catastrophic internal bleeding.

The Science

The discussion on aortic aneurysms is a story of two concurrent truths. IN the first instance, Taiwanese research has indicated that having obstructive sleep apnoea does not increase the risk of subsequent development of an aortic aneurysm unless the patient also has chronic obstructive pulmonary disease (26).

The other truth though, according to research from Switzerland, is that in those who have obstructive sleep apnoea are more likely to have an aortic aneurysm but only in the upper aspect within the chest (thoracia aorta) (27). Further to this, the worse the obstructive sleep apnoea, the greater the likelihood of having such an aneurysm.

8. Asthma

Asthma is a disease of the lungs. It affects the tubes that carry air down from the windpipe. More specifically it affects the medium sized tubes. A patient with asthma will experience shortness of breath and difficulty breathing. There are many triggers for asthma, including having a background of allergic diseases such as hay fever (known as allergic rhinitis) and eczema. Cold air coming in contact with the breathing tubes may also be a trigger for an attack.

During an asthma attack, the walls of the breathing tubes undergo a process of narrowing. This narrowing is caused by the contraction of small muscles that surround the breathing tubes. This contraction results in a squeezing pressure on the breathing tubes, similar to someone putting their hands around someone's neck and strangling them, though on a miniature scale.

The Science

Asthma and obstructive sleep apnoea share some co-existent risk factors and each of these individually are a risk for the other in a reciprocal manner (28). The common pathways of the disease seem to relate to inflammation and neural-immune system interactions. Identifying obstructive sleep apnoea in those with asthma is vital as undiagnosed or untreated obstructive sleep apnoea adversely affects asthma control. The severity of acute asthma attacks is well known to be much worse in those with obstructive sleep apnoea too (29).

The relationship of asthma severity and obstructive sleep apnoea is not just in adults, it also extends into the paediatric age group with the co-existence of the diseases increasing the likelihood that a child will need continuous positive airway pressure therapy to help their obstructed breathing (30)

9. Atrial Fibrillation

The heart has a left and a right-hand side and on each side it is divided into a smaller and larger chamber. The smaller chambers are known as the atria, and the larger ones are called the ventricles. When the heart pumps blood, it needs to move it from the smaller to the larger chamber. This requires a co-ordination of the contraction of the heart muscles.

Starting at the origin point of electrical activity of the heart, there is a focal point known as the atrial node. This initiates a pulse of electrical activity that flows though in built wiring within the heart. This electrical pulse then tells the muscles to contract. If the activity of the atrial node becomes erratic, then instead of an orderly and controlled sequence of muscle contraction, the muscles individually go in to spasm and this then results in the pumping action of the atrium becoming less effective than it should be. This in turn has an impact on blood emptying from the atrium in to the ventricle.

The situation described above is known as atrial fibrillation. With a poorly co-ordinated pumping action, blood ends up filling the chamber of the atrium more than it should due to the continuous flow into the chamber but a deficit in the output. This increase in volume puts pressure on the walls of the atrium and over time they start to be stretched and the heart starts to fatigue and fail.

The Science

Researchers in Norway sought to determine if patients presenting to their clinic with atrial fibrillation also had underlying and undiagnosed obstructive sleep apnoea. The found an extra-ordinary 82% of patients did indeed have obstructive sleep apnoea, and in over half of such patents the severity of disease was significant (31). What was also insightful was that the routine screening questionaries for obstructive sleep apnoea were not at all helpful at identifying underlying airway and sleep pathology.

When it comes to the outcomes of instituting treatments of obstructive sleep apnoea in the context of atrial fibrillation, Chinese clinicians did a meta-analysis of such outcomes in response to the use of continuous positive airway pressure (32). The findings are reassuring in that for those who maintain compliance with therapy, the heart rate irregularities respond favourably.

Muscles work by being stimulated by some form of electrical current. The heart has an intricate level of internal wiring to conduct this electrical pulse. This is necessary to co-ordinate the muscular contractions of the heart in an orderly manner. The first stage of pumping of blood is to move it from the smaller chamber known as the atrium to the bigger chamber known as the ventricle. This means the muscles of the atrium need to contract first, and there needs to be a slight delay before the ventricle starts to pump the blood.

To achieve this, there is, in effect, a form of insulation that means the electrical current conducted through the atrium cannot directly pass to the ventricle in a general manner. Instead, there is a small pathway that the current can pass through from which it is then redistributed through the heart muscle of the ventricle. In effect it is like a delay switch.

The point at which his electrical current is momentarily paused is called the atrioventricular node, or AV node for short. If there is a problem with this node, and the electrical current can not pass through it, then this is known as atrioventricular block. This block in conduction results in a ventricle having to work out for itself when to contract, and often the timing is way off and the heart fails to pump in an adequate way, resulting in heart failure.

The Science

This condition is not a frequently encountered situation, with most of the scientific publications being case reports. An earl case series published in 1977 mentions this type of conductive heart rhythm disorder and how it and others were successfully managed by the only treatment option at the time for obstructive sleep apnoea, a surgically created airway through the windpipe known as a tracheostomy (33).

We have come a long way since then, and given one of the modern treatment options for atrioventricular block is a cardia pacemaker, it is important that underlying obstructive sleep apnoea is not missed as part of the clinical workup of this condition (34). This is important because treatment of the underlying obstructive sleep apnoea may also cure the cardiac arrythmia (35).

11. Attention Deficit Hyperactivity Disorder (ADHD)

There are well defined criteria for the diagnosis of attention deficit hyperactivity disorder. The condition is actually two different types of disease. There is a hyperactivity form and an attention deficit form. An individual may demonstrate one or the other or both forms of symptoms that define the condition.

For the hyperactivity variant, the list of symptoms includes fidgeting hands or feet, squirming in their chair, running about where it is not appropriate, unable to play or take part in leisure activities quietly, talking excessively, trouble waiting their turn, and often interrupting others

For the attention deficit variant, the symptoms include making careless mistakes, seeming to not be listening when spoken to, not following through on instructions, trouble organising tasks, avoiding tasks that require mental effort over a long period of time, easily distracted, and often forgetful in daily activities.

The Science

Way back in 1997 a group of researchers in the Department of Neurology at the University of Michigan Medical Center published research showing children with sleep disordered breathing being misdiagnosed as having AHDH (36). In children who were diagnosed as having ADHD, they were about three times more likely to be snoring and they estimated that 25% of children did not have ADHD in the first place.

In 2007, research from the same university as above sought to determine what level of ADHD actually got better in children treated for their associated airway obstruction (37). Their results were staggering, with not 25% but rather 50% of children having their symptoms resolve to the point that they no longer met the criteria for ADHD.

12. Barret's Oesophagus

The stomach produces a very strong and concentrated form of hydrochloric acid. This acid helps in the digestion process as it breaks down consumed foods in to smaller constituents. The stomach lining is very tough and conditioned to cope with these high acid levels. If it were not, then the acid would end up consuming the stomach itself, an outcome that clearly has unfavourable consequences. When people develop a stomach ulcer, this is exactly part of the process that is occurring.

If a patient suffers from reflux, which is the involuntary passage of stomach contents back up into the oesophagus, this will result in some of the stomach acid washing over the lining of the oesophagus. This acid is very irritating to the lining and this irritation leads to the lining changing its characteristics to become more resilient to the acid damage- a bit like how you develop calluses on your palms with physical labour.

This change in the lining though has a downside, which is that the tissue is prone to damage at a cellular level in the DNA. Such early changes are called Barrett's oesophagus, and this is a prelude to further DNA damage that can result in oesophageal cancer.

The Science

There is a difficult element to researching the impact of obstructive sleep apnoea on the development of Barrett's oesophagus because obstructive sleep apnoea is a risk for reflux and obesity is a risk factor for both reflux and obstructive sleep apnoea. Researchers from the Mayo Clinic sought to clarify this difficult situation and published their results in 2014 (38). They found that having obstructive sleep apnoea increased the chances of progressing to Barrett's oesophagus by 80%. Furthermore, the general risk increased as the severity of the airway obstruction increased. These findings have been confirmed by similar research published in 2020 by the West Virginia University (39).

13. Bedwetting

In medical terminology, bedwetting is known as enuresis. There is a normal phase of childhood development that sees a transition from night time bedwetting to night time control. The is no specific age that defines a cut-off point, but it is possibly generally accepted that this age is about 6-8 years

Ongoing bedwetting can be a source of consternation for the family unit. It places a burden on the need to do regular laundry, causes embarrassment to the child, and also can cause social limitations such as precluding them from having the confidence to do a sleep over at a friend's house.

The normal approach to bedwetting beyond a generally accepted age is consider strategies such as fluid restriction leading up to bed time, the use of night time alarms, and medication. An overlooked contributing factor is upper airway obstruction.

The Science

In February 2018 there was a publication in the Journal of Pediatric Urology by childhood urology specialists that was a systematic review of the literature on whether adenoid and tonsil surgery may help children with bed wetting (40). IN their results they summarise a finding of about 50% of children stopping bed wetting completely and another 20% being better but not perfect.

Coincidentally, research from ENT Specialists in Istanbul was published in the International Journal of Otorhinolaryngology in the same month as the above (41). Once again they found about a 50% resolution rate of bed wetting in children having adenoid and tonsil surgery for upper airway obstruction.

Research findings like the above led to the International Children's Continence Society publishing guidelines in 2020 on looking for underlying causes with upper airway obstruction featuring prominently on the list (42).

14. Benign Prostatic Hyperplasia

This is obviously a disease of men. The prostate is a glandular structure related to the genitourinary tract. It surrounds part of the pluming related to urination, known as the urethra. When the prostate gland enlarges, it reduces the calibre of the urethra which means urinary flow from the bladder through the urethra is compromised. The consequence of this is that men may have trouble passing urine and when they do so the urinary flow is slow, and hence may take quite the while to go to the toilet. The other issue is that the bladder is unable to empty properly, meaning it may take sa man several more trips to the bathroom than normal to achieve adequate emptying of their bladder.

The prostate enlargement is known as benign in this scenario to differentiate it from the other common cause of enlargement which is prostate cancer.

The Science

Research conducted in Taiwan looked at over 1200 men and sought to determine the likelihood of developing benign prostatic hyperplasia within the first 5 years from the diagnosis of obstructive sleep apnoea (43). There results were remarkable for finding a general increased rate of benign prostatic hyperplasia in men over the age of 30 who were diagnosed with obstructive sleep apnoea, at a rate of more than twice the rate of those who did not have obstructive sleep apnoea. Things changed significantly for those who were over the age of 50, with a 5-6 times increased rate of benign prostatic hypertrophy in those with obstructive sleep apnoea.

With such a result, outlined above there is the question as to why this is the case. One concern is that certain medications used for benign prostatic hypertrophy may in turn affect sleep. Indeed, a recent study has confirmed an association between the use of a type of medication for benign prostatic hypertrophy and obstructive sleep apnoea (44). Further research will help us understand these findings.

The full name of this condition is bipolar affective disorder. It is a mental health diagnosis usually made by psychiatrists. The disease has variable elements that make up the diagnosis and also depending on the elements present at any particular stage can have 2 broad manifestations, which is reflected in the name itself.

One pole of the disease is that of depression. The other is that of what is known as mania. Sometimes people refer to it as manic depression. Depression is an altered mood state that results in negative thought, lack of motivation, and a loss of self-worth. Mania is completely the opposite where the individual has lots of energy, if overly bight and cheerful, and exudes confidence and charm. Both extremes are disabling for the mental well being of the individual affected by it.

The Science

Researchers in Columbia has shone the light brightly on the link between bipolar affective disorder and obstructive sleep apnoea (45). In their series of patients, they found a rate of 89% of positive sleep study results for obstructive sleep apnoea; the underlying conditions thought to be contributing to this were obesity and certain medications used for treatment of the mental health condition. It has ben stated that obstructive sleep apnoea is the most common non-mental health illness affecting those with bipolar affective disorder (46).

The research cited above from Columbia was further assessed by a larger study in Taiwan (47). They also confirmed the relationship between obstructive sleep apnoea and bipolar affective disorder, with men being at greater risk, and the confounding factor being the general health of those with mental health problems likely to be affected by obesity.

16. Breast Cancer

Whilst mostly thought to be a disease of women, men too can develop breast cancer. The development of breast cancer is thought to mostly relate to genetics and hormones, with the latter predominantly oestrogen. As this hormone is significantly related to female endocrinology, this helps explain why women are predominantly affected, plus the obvious observation that they have more breast tissue than men, which in turn is more opportunity for something to go wrong.

Apart from the initial development of breast cancer, there are then factors that determine the aggressiveness of the cancers and hence how it may be able to spread. Obstructive sleep apnoea may well play a role in both.

The Science

Korean researchers examined data for over 45,000 women to determine the likelihood of developing breast cancer and how obstructive sleep apnoea may influence the rate of breast cancer development (48). Across all age groups, the diagnosis of obstructive sleep apnoea was associated with a 20% increased his of later development of breast cancer compared to those that dis not have obstructive sleep apnoea. For women over the age of 65 years, this elevated risk was 70%. Research from China has found similar results (49), again about a 2-3 times increased risk of developing breast cancer.

17. Central Serous Chorioretinopathy

The eyeball is a complex system with many intricate parts. It processes a huge amount of information from the environment and to do this has a very high cellular metabolic activity. It is so high that parts of the eye have the highest amount of blood flow per unit weight of tissue in the whole body, with the brain in a close second place. Due to this high metabolic demand, any changes related to oxygen deprivation can often be seen in the eye before any other sign of a problem is evident.

Central serous chorioretinopathy describes the situation where fluid accumulates under the retina, causing it to physically detach from the back of the eye, which results in vision loss. This is something that can be detected by eye specialists using technology known as optical coherence tomography.

The Science

In a meta-analysis of research as of the publication date in 2018, clinicians found that if a patient was found to have central serous chorioretinopathy, there was a 50% increased risk that the patient also had obstructive sleep apnoea (50).

Having identified this association, further research has then sought to clarify what the risk of developing central serous chorioretinopathy is in those that have known obstructive sleep apnoea. Research out of Stanford University suggests that there is indeed an increased risk of the eye condition developing in those with obstructive sleep apnoea (51). Taiwanese research though is even more impressive as they looked at the case files of over 330,000 people (52). They were able to quantify the increased risk of developing central serous chorioretinopathy in those with obstructive sleep apnoea, and this was a 20% increased risk. What was also very helpful was they found that the use of continuous positive airway pressure therapy, that risk was reduced to some degree.

18. Cerebrovascular Disease

This term encompasses the relationship between the blood blow to the brain and the very health of the brain related to this blood flow. In circumstances where there is an issue with the blood flow because of diseases on the blood vessels to the point that it impacts on brain health then this is surmised as being cerebrovascular disease.

The nature of cerebrovascular disease varies depending upon the blood vessels affected and the duration of the problem. Starting from the heart, blood is pumped through major arteries on the neck up to the brain. These blood vessels can become blocked and narrowed, which leads to a reduced amount of blood flow to the brain. The parts of the brain compromised may be specific to the blood vessel that is blocked. The most well-known consequence of a blocked blood vessel is a stroke, where part of the brain dies off due to the lack of blood flow.

From the larger blood vessels, the blood flows into smaller and smaller vessels to reach the brain. If these blood vessels are compromised, it is usually on a global scale that it occurs and hence all of the brain is at risk at the same time. This is what is known as ischaemic microvascular disease.

The Science

With respect to large blood vessels, the prime one of importance are the internal carotid arteries and the vertebral arteries as these are collectively the 4 blood vessels that take blood to the brain, with the former being the most significant. The main pathology that impacts upon these arteries is the development of plaque build up known as atherosclerosis. Research in the United States of America has shown that those with obstructive sleep apnoea were nearly 50% more likely to have plaque build-up in their carotid arteries (53). Researchers mainly based in Poland found that for patients where their plaque build up was so significant that surgery was undertaken to alleviate the blockage, those with obstructive sleep apnoea were twice as likely to need such surgery (54). For patients that end up having a stroke due to the blockage of their large blood vessels, there is once again confirmation of obstructive sleep apnoea increasing the risk of another element of plaque build-up, this being calcium deposition, with South Korean research showing this occurring at a rate that was 18 times that in those with obstructive sleep apnoea compared to those who did not (55).

Apart from the impact on the large blood vessels, the smaller calibre vessels are also compromised n those with obstructive sleep apnoea (56). This leads to deprivation of oxygen to the brain at a regional level and is again associated with smaller forms of strokes. Such damage can lead to dementia too (57).

19. Chipped Teeth and bruxism

Bruxism is the dental term for teeth grinding. The grinding of the teeth may be so significant and severe that the teeth actually start to encounter structural fatigue and start to break or chip away. The act of bruxism can occur when awake and when asleep. Awake bruxism is attribute to psychological to stress most of the time and historically sleep bruxism was attributed to the same

More recent understandings of sleep bruxism have challenged the notion of psychological stress being the full answer to it occurring.

The Science

The debate about the relationship of bruxism to obstructive sleep apnoea is an ongoing one. A recent publication from scientists based mostly in Poland suggests that one reason for bruxism being triggered by obstructive sleep apnoea is that some people have a certain genetic variant in the region involved in coding certain neurotransmitter functions (58).

The other clue as to whether there may be a link between obstructive sleep apnoea is that in some patients the use of continuous positive airway pressure not only alleviates the airway obstruction, but those who had bruxism stopped doing so (59).

A multidisciplinary collaboration by scientists at the Wroclaw Medical University found an association between the presence of obstructive sleep apnoea and bruxism in patients with mild and moderate forms of obstructive sleep apnoea (60). It is curious though that this was not the case with those who have severe obstructive sleep apnoea.

The debate about bruxism and airway obstruction is also not completely resolved, but with research showing parental reports noting the co-existence of the condition, the topic is one certainly worthy of further research (61).

20. Chronic Headaches

Chronic headaches can ruin people's lives. Such headaches come in many shapes and sizes and the common types associated with sleep issues are known as cluster headaches, migraines, tension-type, and a non-specific morning headache. The other cause can be related to jaw joint problems.

For those that are suffering from such headaches, the incapacity can be significant to the point that other pathology such as depression and anxiety start to develop. It is important in any patient afflicted by chronic headaches that any underlying contributing factor is identified.

The Science

There has been a good amount of research investigating the links between headaches and sleep issues for over 10 years at the Center for Sleep Evaluation at the Elliot Hospital, USA (62). The complex relationships between headaches and sleep is becoming better understood through such research.

Over 20 years ago the researchers at the Sleep Disorders Center, Department of Neurology, University of Michigan found that patients suffering from cluster headaches not responding to medication had a remarkable improvement once treatment was instituted for their underlying sleep apnoea (63).

It is interesting to note that children can also suffer from headaches. When it comes to migraines, important research from the Cincinnati Children's Hospital Medical Center has shown a disproportionate amount of sleep disorders in children referred for management of migraines (64). So any way you look at it, for kids and adults alike, those with headaches need to sleep well to be well.

The kidneys are the filters of our blood. Their job is quite complicated as they need to keep a whole range of things in balance. Their tasks include the salt levels in our body, the total fluid levels, removing waste products, regulating blood pressure, and regulating the red blood cell population (important as these carry oxygen throughout our body).

If there is an injury to the kidneys for some reason, they have a certain degree of resilience that is protective but over time if this resilience is eroded, then the kidneys will start to fail. When this happens, then everything listed above can start to be an issue. We can have excess salt building up, excess fluid accumulation, high blood pressure, and anaemia. The problem is that some of these things then become a viscous circle, such as the elevation of blood pressure, which causes more kidney damage. As metabolic waste products will also then build up, patients with chronic kidney failure end up needing dialysis or a transplant to stay alive.

The Science

The fact that about 80% of patients with chronic kidney disease also have obstructive sleep apnoea means that it is essential for patients with kidney disease to have their sleep assessed (65). Obstructive sleep apnoea may worsen chronic kidney disease and may exacerbate high blood pressure.

The relationship between obstructive sleep apnoea and chronic kidney disease is complicated due to the many potential co-existing disease states such as high blood pressure and diabetes, which are both bad for the health of the kidneys, and a recent paper suggests the presence of diabetes in conjunction with obstructive sleep apnoea is more relevant than obstructive sleep apnoea alone for elevating the risk of chronic kidney disease (66). Another complicating factor in patients with both conditions is that the very measurement that determines kidney function is not accurate in those with both conditions (67).

22. Cognitive Impairment

There are many reasons as to why the brain will start to fail. When it comes to sleep and airway, there are many different elements that conspire against brain health.

For starters, we have the issue of airway obstruction leading to reduced oxygen supply to the brain. Another factor is that low oxygen levels induces a state of inflammation which we know is deleterious to the health of all body organs. Another factor is the disturbed sleep patterns interferes with brain activity whilst asleep and this impacts on things like memory and learning. On top of this we have the tiredness and fatigue that comes with poor sleep, with issues that flow on from this such as impaired concentration.

The Science

The brain is surrounded by a circulating layer of fluid known as the cerebrospinal fluid. Spanish and Belgium researchers have tested this fluid for markers of Alzheimer's disease and found that obstructive sleep apnoea is a risk factor for the presence of these markers in the brain fluid (68).

In a collaborative review of the literature, a team of psychiatrists and a respiratory and psychologist found good evidence for concerns about concentration and attention, working memory, episodic memory, and executive functions all being impacted by obstructive sleep apnoea (69).

The problems of brain impairment are not limited to adults. A review of the literature by healthcare professionals in Singapore confirmed the impact of airway obstruction on children (70). With such early damage, there are concerns as to what this then means for the welfare of that child as they develop over time.

23. Decayed Teeth

Dental decay is related to many factors, including sugar in the diet, dental hygiene, fluoride, and possibly genetics. A common factor I the development of dental decay is the action of surface bacteria on the enamel of the teeth. For those people that struggle to breathe through their nose and are hence mouth breathing, there seems to be a change in the bacterial balance of the oral cavity such that bacteria that promote the formation of dental decay are more active.

The Science

As children are more prone to obstruction to nasal airflow, much of the research has been done in this cohort. The findings of a team from the University of Washington and Seattle Children's Hospital is cause for concern (71).

In their protocol, the oral health status was examined clinically and recorded using caries and periodontal indices. They found that children with obstructive sleep apnoea had significantly worse oral health, with the rate of caries 5 times that of the control group. The finding of poor oral health calls for a greater awareness of the importance of healthy breathing.

24. Decreased exercise tolerance

Exercise tolerance refers to how well an individual can endure exercise and also can be assessed by the workload achieved during the exercise period.

Exercise intolerance, therefore, is a reflection of either the inability or decreased ability to perform physical feats at a level that would be normally expected. Exercise intolerance is not an illness as such, but is a reflection of various types of disorders. Such disorders may involve the breathing difficulties, cardiovascular problems, neuromuscular dysfunction, and of course there can be behavioural causes also playing a role.

The Science

Researchers at the University of Sydney in Australia sought to determine the contribution of obstructive sleep apnoea to the exercise tolerance of children that were obese (72). Whist being obese is associated with being in poor physical health, having obstructive sleep apnoea on top of this was the important factor for a reduction in cardiac function during exercise. Not only was this the case, but the more the breathing at night was a problem, reflected in things such as lower oxygen levels for example, the worse the heart was functioning.

An international collaboration of researchers has conducted a meta-analysis of research on this topic as it relates to adults (73). This confirms the link between obstructive sleep apnoea and an altered response of the cardiovascular system to exercise but this is most consistent in those categorised as have severe obstructive sleep apnoea.

25. Decreased Libido

Low libido describes a decreased interest in sexual activity. It can affect both men and women. Low libido may be a reflection of many things, but of concern is that it may be an indicator of an underlying health condition. These could be psychological, such as depression or anxiety, and medical such as low testosterone in men, anaemic, chronic kidney disease and several others. Obstructive sleep apnoea is a significant overlooked cause of decreased libido.

The Science

A published in the Journal of Clinical Sleep Medicine found that men with obstructive sleep apnoea experience lower testosterone levels (74). Combined with the tiredness of poor sleep, this in turn, this leads to decreased libido.

It is not just poor-quality sleep that is the issue. In a study by researchers at the University of Chicago, young, healthy men had their sleep restricted to 5 hours per night for a week (75). Their testosterone levels were decreased by 10 to 15 percent.

Despite the association of obstructive sleep apnoea with decreased libido, the outcomes of treatment with continuous positive airway pressure is not so successful in men, though is quite helpful in women (76). The reasons for this are not fully understood.

26. Dental Malocclusion

When either the teeth, or jaws, or both fail to line up properly, dentists call this a malocclusion. When it is the teeth that are crooked, they call this a dental malocclusion, and when the jaws are crooked, they call it a skeletal malocclusion.

There are many proposed theories as to why the jaws and teeth end up being crooked. Part of the answer seems to lie in genetics and part of the answer seems to lie in environmental factors such as the duration of breast feeding, use of dummies or pacifiers, finger and thumb sucking, and possibly having a breathing problem due to an obstructed upper airway and in particular a blocked nasal breathing pathway. The other interesting aspect of having a malocclusion of the type related to poor jaw development is that underdeveloped jaws can themselves then reduce the amount of space left for the breathing channels and cause airway obstruction.

The Science

The published literature often cites a description of malocclusion in mouth breathing children as "adenoid facies", a term that dates back to 1872 (77). This describes a pattern where the face tends to grow vertically more than it should, and is also hence known as "long face syndrome". This term has subsequently sparked interest and controversy.

In Brazil, researchers had an interest in not only the adenoids, which are anatomical swellings at the back of the nose, but also the tonsils, to see if variations in the size of these impacted on the jaw development (78). In their research, not only did the confirm the suggestion of adenoid facies being a real thing, but also found that large tonsils led to the lower jaw growing forwards more than it should otherwise do so.

27. Depression

Depression is a mental health disease characterised by a low self-esteem, poor motivation, low energy levels, and a low sense of self-worth. It has been associated with altered brain neurochemistry, in particular serotonin. People with depression often feel exhausted, tired, and lacking in energy.

The problem with depression from a symptom point of view is that many are similar to the symptoms attributed to obstructive sleep apnoea, meaning that one condition can be confused for the other, and that if there is dual pathology, one may be missed as an oversight.

The Science

A recent meta-analysis of the literature has confirmed there is more than just an overlap of depression and obstructive sleep apnoea in terms of the nature of symptoms, with untreated obstructive sleep apnoea having an impact on co-existent depression (79).

When it comes to treating obstructive sleep apnoea, in terms of depression, there is research that confirms a definite benefit of using continuous positive airway pressure therapy (80). This benefit, however, is somewhat difficult to measure and be certain of due to the overlapping symptoms of both conditions (81).

So, while there is a general consensus that obstructive sleep apnoea is related to depression, the more recent research has been looking specifically at the impact of obstructive sleep apnoea in pregnant women with respect to manifesting depressive symptoms. In one such study in Australia, the rate of depressive symptoms in pregnant women was increased by a factor of eight if the had obstructive sleep apnoea (82).

28. Diabetes

Diabetes is a medical condition related to the control of blood sugar levels. Normally the blood sugar levels are prevented by going too high by the action of a body hormone called insulin. If there is an inadequate or absence of insulin this is known as type 1 diabetes and the treatment is insulin injections. The other form of diabetes is where the insulin production is adequate, but its effect is limited; this is known as insulin resistance, or type 2 diabetes.

The most common factor leading to type 2 diabetes is obesity. When someone is obese, the response to insulin is blunted, resulting in the bold sugar that should have been cleared from circulation persisting, and hence it becomes elevated. High blood sugar levels have significant consequences in terms of affecting the blood vessels and the neurological system in terms of the brain and nerves.

The Science

Insulin is produced by a body organ known as the pancreas, and specifically by a type of cell known as the "beta cell". While the main reason thought to be causing problems with blood sugar control in those with obstructive sleep apnoea is co-existing obesity, Chines researchers sought to look at the function of these beta-cells to clarify if that is the only factor in play (83). Their study found dysfunctional beta-cell function in those with severe obstructive sleep apnoea.

In terms of the many things that can wrong, Thai researchers focussed on diabetes, kidney function, and atrial fibrillation (all of which are discussed in this book) to determine what problems tended to occur, and they found that of these 3, diabetes was the first medical condition to develop (84).

Once again, with these problems developing, the potential benefit of treatment needs to be clarified. In promising news for those with obstructive sleep apnoea, those treated with continuous positive airway pressure tend to have less diabetes than those not treated (85).

29. Difficult Pregnancy

Pregnancy related conditions include gestational diabetes, gestational hypertension, and gestational reflux. All of these can be transient but ay also be indicative of future problems. The first two of these can also impact on the growth and development of the baby, with impaired growth known as intrauterine growth retardation.

When it comes to pregnancy, the extra weight of the baby can be the tipping balance into developing pregnancy related obstructive sleep apnoea. As highlighted elsewhere in this book, this condition can exacerbate high blood sugar levels, high blood pressure, and reflux. There is a growing interest on the impact of obstructive sleep apnoea on the foetus due to low oxygen levels and all of these other issues that are secondary to the airway obstruction.

The Science

Due to the complex inter-relationship of the conditions listed, the research done on this has been difficult. However, there is some very helpful information coming out.

Starting with high blood pressure, researchers in Japan found that a decrease in the blood oxygen saturation level was a predictor of having high blood pressure later on in the pregnancy (86).

Canadian researchers at the McGill University, focussed on the relationship between sleep disordered breathing and blood glucose levels in women with gestational diabetes (87). In their findings they determined that the worse the co-existing sleep disordered breathing, the higher the blood sugar levels were.

The research on the impact on the foetus is still ongoing.

30. Dry Eye Syndrome

Tears lubricate the eyeball and stops the surface lining from drying out. Every time you blink, a thin film of tears is pushed over the eye surface. This watery layer then has a thinner coat of fatty compounds on the surface of it and this that help to preserve the watery film.

Dry eye syndrome is characterised by insufficient tears. The symptoms include irritation (like having a foreign object in the eye), itchy eyes, and some vision distortion. Over time, the resulting dryness can damage the surface of the eyeball.

The Science

The impact of dry eye syndrome on sleep was highlighted by a review article written by researchers in Japan (88) where they found that sleep quality in those with dry eye syndrome is worse than in other eye disorder. It is so bad that approximately half of patients suffer from poor sleep.

To further explore the topic, scientists from the Netherlands and United Kingdom found a link between dry eye syndrome and many other medical conditions, including obstructive sleep apnoea (89). Many of the other conditions they found associations with also are independently related to obstructive sleep apnoea.

It was research from Turkey, however, that found the best explanation as to the presence of dry eye syndrome in those with obstructive sleep apnoea (90). In their research they found that the small glands in the eye that makes the protective fatty compound are distorted and potentially not working properly.

31. Eczema

Eczema is a very common skin condition that affects both children and adults. People with eczema have skin that becomes dry and easily irritated. Eczema has an underlying allergic component and is associated with hay fever and asthma.

Most treatments for eczema are about avoiding your triggers, use of special soaps, and limiting contact with chlorine from swimming pools.

Eczema causes the sensation of itchiness, which lends itself to scratching, which releases more chemicals that lead to itching. This scratch and itch cycle can cause discomfort, disrupt sleep and affect quality of life.

The Science

Whilst the itchiness and scratching are deleterious to sleep quality, the association with asthma and more so allergic rhinitis leads to a complicated interaction with obstructive sleep apnoea. Researchers in Taiwan have helped identify that children with eczema have a higher risk of obstructive sleep apnoea, with nearly twice the risk compared to controls (91).

The other important research also comes from Taiwan, where they looked at 1,000,000 sets of patient's data (92). By looking at the onset of diagnosis of obstructive sleep apnoea and reviewing the data for the next 5-6 years, they found an approximately 50% increased chance of developing eczema. More importantly they also then made sure that the controlled for things like hay fever and asthma that could have led to incorrect observations being made.

32. Elevated Cholesterol

Cholesterol came onto the radar of the general public a few decades ago, and almost immediately it got a bad rap. Media articles and news stories influenced the mindset of the public to think that cholesterol was bad and it spurned a food industry response to promote no or low cholesterol foods, even though dietary intake of fat, and not cholesterol, is what affects the cholesterol in the body.

Cholesterol is in fact a vital part of the body in terms of building the individual cells that make up the body, but too much in the blood stream is indeed a bad thing. If there is too much of this fatty substance, it can form into a build up known as plaque, which leads to blockages to blood flow through the blood vessels.

Cholesterol is now better understood than when it was first drawn to the attention of the public, and is now broadly divided into "bad cholesterol, known as LDL, and "good cholesterol" known as HDL.

The Science

A multicentre collaboration performed a meta-analysis on the relationship between obstructive sleep apnoea and abnormal blood cholesterol levels (93). They found that in their pooled data of over 18,000 patients, having obstructive sleep apnoea was associated with an elevation in the LDL (bad) cholesterol and a decrease in the HDL (good) cholesterol. Due to the complexities of obesity that can also impact on cholesterol levels, they performed further analysis and found that the LDL levels seemed to be related to the severity of the airway obstruction. Recent research has shown that treating obstructive sleep apnoea with continuous positive airway pressure therapy delivers a beneficial change in the cholesterol levels (94).

An interesting part of this conversation is that in children, having airway obstruction also increases their blood cholesterol and that once they have surgery, these return closer to normal (95). This emphasises the importance of early treatment to mitigate against potential lifelong cardiovascular disease.

33. Epilepsy

Epilepsy is a common brain disease, with as a tendency to having repeated seizures. The seizures are caused by abnormal electrical activity in the brain. It is estimated that about 1 in every 30 people will experience epilepsy, and it is more likely to start happening in the extremes of age, namely childhood and senior years.

There are many different types of epilepsy and depending on the type, it may be self-limiting it may be a life-long condition. The main form of treatment is medication. The known causes of epilepsy include brain trauma from a physical injury, damage to the brain from a stroke, meningitis, brain tumours, and prolonged oxygen deprivation to the brain.

The Science

There has long been a question of whether having temporary low oxygen levels caused by obstructed breathing at night could exacerbate epilepsy. Researchers in India undertook a literature review of the current evidence and found that the current research is conflicting and contradictory (96). On the one hand, there is an observed rate of co-existent airway obstruction and sleep apnoea, but at the same time there is no clear explanation as to why. One theory is that it may be subtle and brief drops in the brain oxygen levels, rather than substantial and prolonged oxygen drops that lead to increased seizure activity (97). There is still more research needed to fully explain this situation.

In discussing the relationship between epilepsy and obstructive sleep apnoea, an interesting additional observation is that for epilepsy, a certain treatment known as a "Vagus nerve stimulator", which is a surgically implanted device, can cause airway obstruction, probably by inadvertently causing the muscles of the throat to contract and close the airway (98).

34. Erectile Dysfunction

Erectile dysfunction is the medical term for what is more generally known as male impotence. It is not unusual for men to have moments where they are impotent, often related to stress, anxiety, or inebriation with alcohol, but frequent and prolonged impotence may be a sign of an underlying medical condition.

In approaching the condition, three is a significant list of causes that need to be considered, such as cardiovascular disease, diabetes, high blood pressure, obesity, low testosterone, mental health and well-being, sleep disorders, and smoking.

The Science

The list of conditions that may impact on male sexual function clearly has a strong link to obstructive sleep apnoea due to the many associated conditions linked in with this disease. This is conformed by a review carried out by French scientists (99). The question though, is whether treatment of obstructive sleep apnoea can deliver any benefits with so many other potential things also going on that can impact on men achieving an erection. In what should be a favourable motivating outcome to pursue treatment for obstructive sleep apnoea, there are a good number of papers showing improved sexual function with the use of continuous positive airway pressure therapy in men with obstructive sleep apnoea (100) (101) (102).

35. Excessive Daytime Sleepiness

It is not unusual to have the occasional day where you feel sleepy or tired. For those that have this feeling on a consistent and persistent basis, however, may have an underlying sleep disorder. Falling asleep when they should not be, such as in a meeting, at a conference, on a train or bus or even as the driver of a car are typical examples.

Excessive daytime sleepiness affects an estimated 20 percent of the population. Due to the risk of motor vehicle and work-related accidents, it was these problems that first drew the medical community's attention to obstructive sleep apnoea.

The Science

Day time sleepiness is now the foundation of one of the most utilised screening tools, known as the "Epworth sleepiness scale". This was developed and then shared with the world in 1991 by Dr Johns from the Sleep Disorders Unit of the Epworth Hospital in Australia (103). It is a questionnaire that looks at the likelihood of someone falling asleep in eight common day time scenarios: talking to someone, driving a car, the hours after lunchtime, watching television, passenger in a car, reading, sitting in a public place, and seeking to have a lie down in the middle of the afternoon.

Those afflicted by obstructive sleep apnoea should be relieved that the progress in management of obstructive sleep apnoea for excessive day time somnolence has come a long way from when the main surgical option was a tracheostomy, a procedure where a window is made in the windpipe and a person is then breathing through a tube placed through the front of the neck into this window (104).

36. Fibromyalgia

Fibromyalgia is a chronic condition, causing pain in the muscles and bones. In fact, it is the second most common chronic condition affecting the musculoskeletal system. Despite being so common, it is often misdiagnosed because its symptoms mimic those of other conditions. There are also no real tests to confirm the diagnosis. It is theorised that the condition may in part be due to overactive pain perception.

The Science

The potential link between obstructive sleep apnoea and fibromyalgia has been a challenge as the symptoms of fibromyalgia also include fatigue, tiredness and poor sleep, symptoms akin to obstructive sleep apnoea. In trying to delve into this challenge, researchers in Turkey found that 50% of patients with fibromyalgia also had obstructive sleep apnoea (105). Furthermore though, they also found a relationship between the degree of oxygen desaturation and increasing degree of symptoms.

Further research from Turkey has then focussed specifically on women, who for some reason are more prone to fibromyalgia and less prone to obstructive sleep apnoea (106). They found a staggering 65% of women with fibromyalgia also had obstructive sleep apnoea.

37. Floppy Eyelid Syndrome

Floppy eyelid syndrome is a common eye disorder and describes when the eyelid loses elasticity and becomes lax and is easily turned upward. There are variable symptoms, which include irritation and itching of the eyes, especially upon waking. This condition leads to corneal and conjunctival compromise due t exposure to the air by the eyelid lifting up on itself.

The Science

Obstructive sleep apnoea may contribute to local eyelid ischaemia which may play a role in development of floppy eyelid syndrome. Research on this has shown that the more severe the obstructive sleep apnoea is, the more likely it is to have floppy eyelid syndrome (107).

To explore this association further, researchers in Portugal sought to determine if the condition was potentially reversible by using continuous positive airway pressure treatment (108). In a promising outcome, more than half of their patients had the floppy eyelid syndrome resolve after 6 months of therapy. Those with more severe airway compromise were less likely to show such improvements.

38. Glaucoma

Glaucoma is an eye disease that has four different forms and is important because it causes irreversible vision loss due to damage to the optic nerve. The damage is often caused by an abnormally high pressure in the eye.

Glaucoma can occur at any age but is more common in older adults.

The Science

The relationship between obstructive sleep apnoea and certain types of glaucoma is of interest to eye specialists as the presence of one condition has been suggested to seek out if the other is also present (109). Having said that though, not all types of glaucoma have a relationship to obstructive sleep apnoea and the relationship to the normal measurement of a sleep study known as the apnoea-hypopnoea index is not entirely straightforward (110).

When continuous positive airway pressure therapy is employed in treating patients who have obstructive sleep apnoea and glaucoma, the findings are interesting as the pressure levels in the eye seem to persist but the visual loss does not (111). This raises the possibility that there is more than one reason for the co-existence of the disease, or that the pressure therapy is not completely eliminating some of the pathological processes.

39. Growth impairment

In children, it has long been recognised that those with trouble breathing at night tend to smaller in stature. There are many reasons for why this may well be the case. At a basic level having airway obstruction affects the appetite, with children tending to eat less as a result. Children also tend to have an increased metabolic rate if they have upper airway obstruction, in part due to the increased effort involved in breathing to overcome the obstruction. Another physical element is that large tonsils lead to swallowing problems, which means dietary intake may be impacted.

Apart from the physical elements outlined above, possibly a more significant issue in children with upper airway obstruction is that the regulation of growth hormone release is impacted in children with sleep disordered breathing.

The Science

Spanish researchers and surgeons collaborated in 2018 to assess for growth retardation in children with obstructive sleep apnoea, and to monitor subsequent growth patterns once children had surgery for their obstruction (112). They confirmed that children with airway obstruction tended to be smaller both in terms of height and weight. Once surgery was done, 12 months after, about two thirds of the children had achieved a size and weight comparable to their peers.

One of the proposed mechanisms of growth retardation is an impairment in growth hormone activity, and as this hormone exerts its effect via a mediator known as "insulin-like growth factor", research has focussed on whether there any measurable changes in the activity of this mediator. Turkish research would suggest that there is indeed an issue with growth hormone activity, as children have altered levels of insulin like growth factor if they have obstructed breathing, and improvements follow once they have surgery (113) (114).

Our bodies are full of colonies of harmless bacteria. In fact, there are trillions of microorganisms in the gastrointestinal tract. Most of these bacteria make a positive contribution to our health by promoting food digestion, facilitation our metabolism, and regulation exerting an influence on the immune system.

Dysbiosis describes the situation where there is an imbalance in the types of gut bacteria. A persistent imbalance of is associated with inflammatory bowel diseases, cancer, diabetes, obesity, cardiovascular disease and brain function.

The Science

Due to the complexities of gut dysbiosis, much of the research thus far is done using animal models. Scientific research from California looked at the impact of low oxygen and high carbon dioxide levels (which are the consequence of airway obstruction) in mice and conformed a change in the gut bacteria ecology (115).

The concern about gut dysbiosis is that is seems to contribute to certain metabolic and systemic health issues, a theory that was supported in 2019 by researchers in China (116). A systemic literature review confirmed the relationship between gut dysbiosis and the development of high blood pressure too (117).

An interesting new piece of information that is still in the category of emerging understanding is that the gut microbiome may actually exert some form of control over breathing itself (118) and that changes in the microbiome may be a risk factor for colon cancer (119).

41. Hearing Loss

There are many reasons for losing hearing, and most people tend to put it down to old age in adults and ear infections in children. There are a range of ways that snoring and sleep apnoea could theoretically impact on the hearing too.

The Science

In children, those with upper airway obstruction have an increased chance of having a build up of fluid in their middle ear spaces, which will then lead to a hearing loss (120).

In adults, there seems to be a different pathway to hearing loss. For example, it is reasonable to suggest that the noise of snoring itself may impact on the hearing due to prolonged exposure t the noise resulting in damage. This theory would seem to be supported as they type of hearing loss that would develop is one that impacts on the higher frequencies, which is exactly what scientific research in Turkey confirms (121). This finding is supported by other research from China, but interestingly they also detected subtle changes in the activity of the nerve that then carries sound from the inner ear to the brain (122).

Unfortunately, contrary to many things that seem to get better once an adult starts using positive airway pressure therapy, the hearing seems to continue to be a problem with respect to hearing loss (123).

42. High Blood Pressure

As blood is pumped by the heart around the body, the pressure of the blood goes up and down as the heart contracts and then relaxes. When blood pressure is measured, it is reflective of the highest reading (systolic blood pressure) and the lowest reading (diastolic blood pressure). Blood pressure is traditionally measured relative to the historical way of measuring pressure, which was the displacement of the element Mercury within a tube; this is written as a number followed by the unit of measurement which is "mmHg".

The blood pressure is high if the reading is higher than 140 for the systolic and/or 90 mmHg for the diastolic. Elevated blood pressure increases the risk of having a heart attack or stroke High blood pressure is known as hypertension.

The Science

There is growing evidence of the causal link between upper airway obstruction and the development of high blood pressure, including an understanding on the mechanisms leading to this latter condition developing (124) (125). In identifying this relationship, one of the historical issues that complicates the discussion is that there have been different ways of defining adult obstructive sleep apnoea, and in doing so, this affects the diagnosis and then the identified relationship to high blood pressure (126). By having a more inclusive diagnosis, more patients fall into the category of having obstructive sleep apnoea. This is important because research shows a benefit to managing high blood pressure in those diagnosed with obstructive sleep apnoea (127).

When it comes to children, there is also some evidence of early vascular changes associated with the development of high blood pressure and cardiovascular disease (128). In somewhat concerning research findings, patients who had upper airway obstruction as children were much more likely to then be diagnosed with high blood pressure within a ten-year time frame (129).

43. Hypercoagulable Disorder

When you bleed, and the blood clots, this is called coagulation. This is a normal process, but sometimes there can be a situation when the blood starts to clot when it should not, and this may be referred to as a hypercoagulable state. Abnormally forming blood clots may result n a problem with blood then flowing through the blood vessel to its intended destination. The blood clots may also break off and travel to other parts of the body. This can result in death of body

The Science

There are many reasons for the blood clotting more than it should, and this includes overactivity of the protein clotting factors and the blood components known as platelets. In obstructive sleep apnoea, these are both an issue (130).

In terms of quantifying the magnitude of risk, a meta-analysis in 2015 suggested there was a two to three times risk of a patient with obstructive sleep apnoea developing some form of abnormal blood clot (131). Research from South Africa suggests the time it takes to develop a hypercoagulable state is no more than three years (132). IN good news though, Italian research has shown that one month of continuous positive airway pressure therapy for one month can start to bring about a return to normal values (133).

44. Hypothyroidism

The thyroid gland is located in the lower front portion of the neck. It creates a hormone known as thyroxine. This hormone is responsible for providing a stimulus to to nearly every organ in your body. It affects functions like the heart beating and how the digestive system moves its contents along. If there is a diminished level of thyroxine, known as hypothyroidism, the body's processes will start to slow down.

In the early stages, hypothyroidism may not cause noticeable symptoms. Over time though, people start to put on weight, feel lethargic and tired, and notice they can not think as clearly as they used to.

The Science

The similarity of symptoms of poor sleep of obstructive sleep apnoea and hypothyroidism should clearly highlight the need to consider each condition with the presenting symptoms tiredness. The problem is that hypothyroidism can directly cause obstructive sleep apnoea and also exacerbate the metabolic consequences of upper airway obstruction (134). In this cited study, they found a rate of thyroid dysfunction to be 16% and half of that fell into the sub-clinical category, meaning the thyroid function was decreased, but the patients were not yet manifesting symptoms directly attributable to the low thyroid function. Research from the USA in over 5,000 patients found this rate to be over 10%, so again it highlights just how common the thyroid dysfunction is in those struggling to breathe properly at night (135).

45. Irritable Bowel Syndrome

Irritable bowel syndrome is one of the most frequent gastrointestinal afflictions. It decreases quality of life of those afflicted by the condition, with symptoms such as abdominal pain, bloating, altered bowel habit, and flatulence.

The cause of irritable bowel syndrome is not well understood. Having said that though, there are some factors that have been identified that seem to play a role. These include a change in the gut bacteria profile, inflammation of the tissue of the bowel, and stress and anxiety.

There is no known cure and therapy centres around diet, counselling, and relaxation exercises.

The Science

Research conducted at the sleep laboratory at the Isfahan University of Medical Sciences demonstrated a link between sleep apnoea and irritable bowel syndrome (136). In fact, there was a nearly 400% increased rate of irritable bowel disease in those with obstructive sleep apnoea compared to those who did not have obstructive sleep apnoea.

One of the other issues with irritable bowel syndrome is that it impacts upon sleep quality in its own right, resulting in sleep fragmentation and tiredness during the day (137). This is another example of a vicious circle that can develop. Fortunately for suffers of both obstructive sleep apnoea and irritable bowel syndrome, the literature suggests the use of CPAP can have a beneficial effect in controlling both conditions (138).

46. Leg Cramps at Night

Leg cramps at night are particularly common, with up to 60% of adults having at least one episode of waking in the middle of the night due to the pain. Whilst this condition is widespread, its causes and cures are uncertain. This uncertainty means that those rare causes that are amenable to management may be missed by a treating medical doctor.

The Science

In keeping with the sparse details on leg cramps, the science on its relationship is negligible. There are however several case reports suggesting that continuous positive airway pressure in those experiencing leg cramps in the context of having obstructive sleep apnoea resulted in a resolution of the painful night time disruptions to sleep (139).

47. Low Testosterone

These two words together seem to strike fear into the hearts (and elsewhere) of men. Low testosterone is a cause of significant symptoms, and these include reduced libido, fatigue, loss of muscle mass, irritability, erectile dysfunction, and depression. With such symptoms, it is not unusual that men will seek out a management strategy if they have ow testosterone, and this includes taking supplement testosterone therapy.

The Science

The relationship between low testosterone and obstructive sleep apnoea is a rather complex one. On one hand, having obstructive sleep apnoea may well be associated with low testosterone, on the other hand treating the low testosterone with a supplement may make the obstructive sleep apnoea worse (140).

Whilst the presence of both obstructive sleep apnoea and low testosterone is noted, the attribution of the low testosterone to the airway obstruction may be misplaced, with research showing that obesity is more the issue for those with low testosterone (141). This would then also explain the observation that continuous positive airway pressure makes no difference to the testosterone levels (142). This emphasises that for those with both conditions, independent management would be appropriate, and where being overweight is a factor, addressing this has mutual benefit to each condition.

48. Melanoma

Melanoma is a serious form of skin cancer that begins in the skin's pigment cells known as melanocytes. Melanoma is a dangerous form of skin cancer. It grows very quickly if left untreated. It can enter the lymphatic system or bloodstream and then spread to other parts of the body such as the lungs, liver, brain and bones.

The best results for melanoma is with early detection and removal. In the event of aggressive disease, then more extensive surgery together with radiotherapy, chemotherapy, and immunotherapy may be necessary.

The Science

Epidemiological research has suggested that obstructive sleep apnoea is associated with certain types of cancer, including melanoma (143). The mechanisms as to why this may be the case have been the subject of research.

In 2018 a publication by researchers from Spain started to help explain the underlying pathology (144). In their study they found that a certain marker involved in blood vessel development was higher in those with obstructive sleep apnoea. Chinese researchers using an animal model confirmed that the body responses that follow on from low oxygen levels were also implicated in the disease (145).

In 2019 the Spanish research group fond even more reasons as to why melanoma was worse in those with obstructive sleep apnoea (146).

49. Multiple Sclerosis

Multiple sclerosis is a disease of the central nervous system, interfering with nerve impulses within the brain and spinal cord. The disease process, in simple terms, is that the immune system attacks myelin, which is the protective layer around nerve fibres. When this protective layer is lost, nerve cells are no longer able to send their electrical pulses in an effective manner. Multiple sclerosis causes many different symptoms, including loss of vision, pain, fatigue and impaired motor function. The symptoms, severity and duration vary from one person to the next.

Whilst there is currently no known cure for multiple sclerosis, there are a number of management options which help manage symptoms and slow the progression of the disease.

The Science

Whilst there is disagreement as to what proportion of patients with multiple sclerosis also have upper airway obstruction, the general consensus is that the rate of breathing problems is high n those with multiple sclerosis than those without it (147). The concern about obstructive sleep apnoea in patients with multiple sclerosis is that the latter disease may affect the parts of the brain that control breathing, and the former disease may induce an inflammatory response which exacerbates the immune system mediated damage to the nervous system.

50. Nocturia

Nocturia is the medical term for waking up at night and having to pass urine. Whilst it may be common for people to experience this as they get older, underlying causes need to be considered as the sleep disturbance brought about by trips to the bathroom can have a delirious impact on health and well-being.

The Science

A literature review published in 2020 found that having obstructed breathing when asleep increased the likelihood of additional sleep disturbances by nocturia in men but not in women (148). This research though, tended to reflect an older population group, in which there could be other factors at play. In research of young adults, the link between obstructed breathing and nocturia has been demonstrated, and it is therefore important for young adults that do not have any risk factors for nocturia be screened for an airway problem (149). The same applies to patients with other urinary symptoms such as incontinence (150).

An important consideration with obstructed breathing and nocturia is whether the treatment of the upper airway obstruction also translates into a reduction in the need to get up and go to the bathroom. In good news for patients, some research showed that about half of patients had a reduced need to get up and urinate at night (151).

While it is normal for there to be some fat in the liver, if more than 5-10% of the liver's weight is fat, then it is called a fatty liver. Non-alcoholic fatty liver disease is the build-up of excess fat in cells of liver that is not caused by alcohol. If the condition progresses, it can lead to marked inflammation of the liver and potentially liver failure.

Unfortunately, the cause of non-alcoholic fatty liver disease is unknown but identified risk factors include obesity, high cholesterol, and type 2 diabetes.

The Science

The stated risk factors and known association of these risk factors with upper airway obstruction would lead to the suggestion that non-alcoholic fatty liver disease is a likely outcome in patients with upper airway obstruction. IN a literature of the topic published in 2020, the concerning finding was that non-alcoholic fatty liver disease was more prevalent in those with obstructive sleep apnoea even in the absence of the other risk factors (152). This review also showed that the liver disease was worse as the upper airway obstruction severity increased.

This disease process does not seem to be confined to adults. In a meta-analysis of paediatric publications on the topic, also published in 2020, it was found that having obstructive sleep apnoea as a child also caused derangement of liver function and evidence of disease progress to scarring of the liver (153).

In disappointing news for those with obstructive sleep apnoea, the use of continuous positive airway pressure does not seem to reverse the disease process, with weight loss proving to be far more important (154).

52. Non-arteritic Anterior Ischaemic Optic Neuropathy

The optic nerve is the neurological communication of the eye to the brain. This nerve has a critical blood supply. Non-arteritic anterior ischemic optic neuropathy refers to loss of blood flow to this nerve. This typically results in sudden vision loss in one eye, without any pain. In many cases, the loss of vision in one eye is upon waking up in the morning. Once this happens, the vision usually does not improve.

The exact mechanism causing reduced blood flow to the optic nerve is known to occur more often when a patient has diabetes, high blood pressure, and sleep apnoea.

The Science

Non-arteritic anterior ischaemic optic neuropathy is very rare. This creates the challenge for determining where disease states may be associated, as a large number of cases are needed to be convinced the association is real. Fortunately, Korea maintains an extensive database of health conditions and in a review conducted where they screened over one million patient files, they found enough cases of non-arteritic anterior ischaemic optic neuropathy to relate this condition to obstructive sleep apnoea, with the finding being a subsequent increased risk of the eye disease in those with a new diagnosis obstructive sleep apnoea (155).

A similar designed study in Taiwan showed the risk of developing non-arteritic anterior ischaemic optic neuropathy doubles if someone is diagnosed with obstructive sleep apnoea (156).

A helpful situation in the scenario of a patient facing possible visual loss would be signs of early disease before it gets to the visual loss stage. Fortunately, there are early signs of compromise to the blood flow to the optic nerve that a specialised eye assessment can detect (157).

53. Overactive Bladder Syndrome

Overactive bladder syndrome is not a disease but rather is the terminology used to describe a group of urinary symptoms. It characterised by an increased frequency to urinate together with incontinence and frequent awakening periods during night time to go to the bathroom.

It is estimated that 30-40 percent% of people are affected to some degree. Many of these people living do not ask for help. The symptoms at night time can disrupt sleep quality due to frequent trips to the toilet.

There are many myths about this condition, such as it normal part of getting older, it just part of being a woman, and it an issue related to the prostate in men.

Historically, treatments to help people manage their symptoms include lifestyle changes such as limiting fluid intake before going to bed, medications, botulinum toxin injections, nerve stimulation devices, and surgery.

There are treatments to help even minor OAB symptoms.

The Science

For some time, the issue of interrupted sleep due to overactive bladder syndrome has been noted. In more recent times the question has been raised as to whether obstructive sleep apnoea could be causing some of the issues. To explore this further, researchers from the Hospital del Mar in Barcelona, Spain, analysed female patients referred to a sleep disorders clinic with suspected sleep apnoea (158). All patients completed a questionnaire their bladder control relating to the feeling of urgency to urinate, frequency of urination, incontinence and nocturnal urination. They found that women with obstructive sleep apnoea higher scores for the prevalence of symptoms associated with bladder control and their discomfort with these symptoms.

Having made this link, the next question that needs answering is whether treatment of obstructive sleep apnoea also helps the urinary symptoms. Researchers in Turkey have investigated this and it seems that the answer to this question is that indeed it does help (159). This is very significant as it suggests that there may be unnecessary medical or interventional treatment still being conducted in such patients.

54. Parkinson's Disease

Parkinson's disease is a progressive neurological condition degenerative that affects the control of body movements. It causes a host of varying symptoms, such as trembling of the hands, arms, legs, jaw, and face and stiffness of the limbs and trunk, together with slow of body movements and unstable posture resulting in difficulty with walking.

Parkinson's disease is linked to the slow death of nerve cells that produce a neurotransmitter known as dopamine. Dopamine is important as the messenger for relaying messages between areas of the brain that control body movement. When the dopamine levels are low, there is difficulty in controlling muscle function.

So far, scientists have not determined the reason why some people develop Parkinson's disease and others do not.

The Science

The relationships between sleep disturbances and Parkinson's disease are complex and not well understood. A systemic review did, however, confirm that sleep is definitely an issue for those with Parkinson's disease and that obstructive sleep apnoea is an element of the sleep issues (160).

One treatment for Parkinson's disease is to elevate the dopamine levels using a medication known as Levo-dopa. In one research study the more this medication was used, the more it seemed to have a protective effect in lessening obstructive sleep apnoea (161).

In what is of great importance is that the standard treatments of obstructive sleep apnoea deliver benefits to those with Parkinson's disease except for the motor dysfunctions, highlighting the need to be comprehensive in managing patients with both conditions (162).

55. Periodontal Disease

Periodontal disease is better known as gum disease. The disease is caused initially by bacteria building up on the teeth which we all call plaque. The plaque that is not removed with brushing and flossing can lead to sore, bleeding gums, pain on chewing, and tooth loss in worse case scenarios.

In the advanced stages of periodontal disease, only professional cleaning by a dentist or dental hygienist can remove the plaque build-up. Sometimes this involves cleaning the pockets around teeth to prevent damage to surrounding bone.

The Science

Children are more prone to upper airway obstruction, and in such children research has shown more periodontal disease, more sites of such disease within the mouth ff such children, and more severe disease when compared to normal breathing children (71).

This association has been subject to much research and in more recent times there is a growing understanding that having obstructive sleep apnoea leads to stimulation of inflammatory pathways that are common to the disease process of periodontitis, and this then exacerbates the latter (163).

56. Polycystic Ovary Syndrome

Polycystic ovary syndrome is a hormonal disorder which may affect women of reproductive age. The hormonal changes may include excess male hormone production, irregular menstrual periods, and difficulty with conceiving. Associated with this condition, in 80% of cases, there is also insulin resistance, a forerunner to diabetes. It is suggested that up to 70% of cases go undiagnosed.

The Science

In a nationwide longitudinal follow-up study using the Taiwan National Health Insurance Research Database, women with polycystic ovary syndrome had a 70% increased risk of developing obstructive sleep apnoea than in women without the condition (164). When other potential contributing factors were accounted for, the specific increased risk due to obstructive sleep apnoea alone was a 160%. One meta-analysis has suggested that about one third or women with polycystic ovary syndrome have obstructive sleep apnoea (165).

As each condition in its own right leads to a deceased quality of life, it is of no surprise that research from the United Kingdom shoed co-existing polycystic ovary syndrome and obstructive sleep apnoea led to worse quality of life scores than in those with polycystic ovary syndrome alone (166).

Psychosis is a symptom, not an illness. It describes a situation where the way your brain processes information is disturbed, losing touch with reality. Common experiences are hallucinations, where things may be seen, heard, or even felt when there is nothing to account for that experience. There may also be disordered though processes, with false beliefs such as feeling god-like, being under the influence and control of others, or other delusional thoughts. Psychotic episodes are not uncommon with Australian data suggesting 1 in 200 people every year will experience an episode.

Psychosis may be related to a mental illness, such as schizophrenia, bipolar disorder or severe depression, be induced by drug abuse, or less commonly in response to a stressful event. Lack of sleep is also implicated in the condition manifesting.

The Science

There is limited research on the interaction between having upper airway obstruction and the manifestation of psychosis (167). In fact, the pervading complacency when it comes to healthcare and sleep is exemplified in their findings with less than 10% of patients treated according to clinical guidelines of managing sleep disorders.

This complacency is disappointing when it comes to mental health, because sleep has been shown to impact mental well-being. In reference to psychosis, sleep disorders of many types, not just upper airway obstruction, are associated are predictive of repeated episodes of psychosis (168).

58. Schizophrenia

Schizophrenia is a serious mental health condition. Affected patients may experience hallucinations, delusions, and express these through dysfunctional behaviour. People with schizophrenia struggle to function normally, often neglecting their personal hygiene, lack normal emotional responses to situations, and can be quite withdrawn from society.

Patients with schizophrenia are known to have additional health problems that are a consequence of a poor level of functioning, such as obesity from poor diet and lack of exercise, cardiovascular disease, and diabetes.

The Science

Taiwanese research has identified that patients with schizophrenia are at a greater risk for having obstructive sleep, independent of other health conditions that can overlap in people with both schizophrenia and obstructive sleep apnoea (169).

With both obstructive sleep apnoea and schizophrenia characterised by impaired cognitive thinking, and hence confusing the clinical presentation as to what is causing the problem, the benefit of treating upper airway obstruction with positive airway pressure may indicate that some of the symptoms traditionally attributed to schizophrenia may be manifestations of other pathology (170).

Autoimmune diseases are a type of medical condition where the immune system mounts a response to itself. Some autoimmune diseases target one body part, and others can have a wide affect on many parts of the body Systemic lupus erythematosus is an autoimmune condition which affects the skin, joints, outer lining of the lungs and heart, kidneys, blood cells, and brain.

Most patients with systemic lupus erythematosus have a mild form of the disease, but in rare cases it is life threatening. For those with severe disease, identifying any underlying contributing factor is paramount to management.

The Science

Upper airway obstruction is known to induce an inflammatory response within the body, and it is only in the past 10 years that researchers started to investigate if this inflammation may be implicated in those with autoimmune disease (171). IN the first published study, researchers suggested that there was in increased risk of developing autoimmune conditions by a factor of nearly double the rate in those with obstructive sleep apnoea compared to those without.

Since this preliminary finding, further research and debate about the association persists (172). In more contemporary research, in patients with obstructive sleep apnoea were found to have elevated blood markers associated with developing autoimmune diseases and these inflammatory markers are then normalised in patients on continuous positive airway pressure, so while there is no definite explanation, scientists are starting to get a better understanding on this still uncertain relationship (173).

References

1. *On Some Causes of Backwardness and Stupidity in Children: And the Relife of these Symptoms in Some Instances by Naso-Pharyngeal Scarifications.* **Hill, W.** s.l. : Br Med J, 1889 Sep 28; 2(1500): 711–712.

2. *Neurobehavioral Outcomes in School-Aged Children with Primary Snoring.* **Hagström K, et al.** s.l. : Arch Clin Neuropsychol, 2020;35(4):401-412.

3. *Parent report of children's sleep disordered breathing symptoms and limited academic progress in reading, writing, and math.* **Harding R, et al.** s.l. : Sleep Med, 2020;65:105-112.

4. *Sleep disordered breathing symptoms and daytime sleepiness are associated with emotional problems and poor school performance in children.* **Liu J, et al.** s.l. : 2016;242:218-225, Vol. Psychiatry Res.

5. *Sleep Disordered Breathing and Academic Performance: A Meta-analysis.* **Galland B, et al.** s.l. : Pediatrics, 2015;136(4):e934-e946.

6. *Gastroesophageal reflux disease is associated with high risk of obstructive sleep apnea syndrome.* **Chen Y, et al.** s.l. : Zhonghua Nei Ke Za Zhi, 2018 Nov 1;57(11):824-829.

7. *Correlation of sleep-disordered breathing and laryngopharyngeal reflux: a two-channel triple-sensor pHmetry catheter study.* **Erdem D, et al.** s.l. : Eur Arch Otorhinolaryngol, 2018 Oct;275(10):2585-2592.

8. *Laryngopharyngeal reflux in obstructive sleep apnoea patients: Literature review and meta-analysis.* **Magliulo G, et al.** s.l. : Am J Otolaryngol, 2018 Nov-Dec;39(6):776-780.

9. *The relationship between obstructive sleep apnea hypopnea syndrome and gastroesophageal reflux disease: a meta-analysis.* **Wu ZH, et al.** s.l. : Sleep Breath, 2019 Jun;23(2):389-397.

10. *Effect of continuous positive airway pressure on gastroesophageal reflux in patients with obstructive sleep apnea: a meta-analysis.* **Li C, et al.** s.l. : Sleep Breath, 2020 Oct 28. doi: 10.1007/s11325-020-02224-9.

11. *Relationship between reflux diseases and obstructive sleep apnea together with continuous positive airway pressure treatment efficiency analysis.* **Wang L, et al.** s.l. : Sleep Med, 2020 Aug 5;75:151-155.

12. *Sleepless in America: inadequate sleep and relationships to health and well-being of our nation's children.* **Smaldone A, et al.** s.l. : Pediatrics, 2007 Feb;119 Suppl 1:S29-37.

13. *Nighttime sleep duration and externalizing behaviors of preschool children.* **Scharf RJ, et al.** s.l. : J Dev Behav Pediatr, 2013 Jul-Aug;34(6):384-91.

14. *Event-related potentials and behavior performance scores in children with sleep-disordered breathing.* **Kaihua J, et al.** s.l. : Brain Dev, 2019 Sep;41(8):662-670.

15. *Aggressive behavior, bullying, snoring, and sleepiness in schoolchildren.* **O'Brien LM, et al.** s.l. : Sleep Med, 2011 Aug;12(7):652-8.

16. *The Relationship Between Obstructive Sleep Apnea and Alzheimer's Disease.* **Andrade AG, et al.** s.l. : J Alzheimers Dis, 2018;64(s1):S255-S270, J Alzheimers Dis.

17. *Obstructive Sleep Apnoea and Alzheimer's Disease: In Search of Shared Pathomechanisms.* **Polsek D, et al.** s.l. : Neurosci Biobehav Rev, 2018 Mar;86:142-149, Neurosci Biobehav Rev.

18. *Sleep-dependent Memory Consolidation in Healthy Aging and Mild Cognitive Impairment.* **Pace-Schott EF, Spencer RMC.** s.l. : Curr Top Behav Neurosci, 2015;25:307-30, Curr Top Behav Neurosci.

19. *Sleep-disordered Breathing Advances Cognitive Decline in the Elderly.* **Osorio RS, et al.** s.l. : Neurology, 2015 May 12;84(19):1964-71, Neurology.

20. *Hypoxemia During Sleep and the Progression of Coronary Artery Calcium.* **Seo MY, et al.** s.l. : Cardiovasc Toxicol, 2020;10.1007/s12012.

21. *Undiagnosed sleep apnoea in cardiac rehabilitation: Age-dependent effect on diastolic function in coronary artery disease patients with preserved ejection fraction.* **Alonderis A, et al.** s.l. : Eur J Cardiovasc Nurs, 2020;1474515120941373.

22. *Risk factors of coronary artery stenosis in patients with obstructive sleep apnoea: a prospective study.* **Wan Y, et al.** s.l. : J Pak Med Assoc, 2019;69(11):1610-1616.

23. *The common denominators of sleep, obesity, and psychopathology.* **Tubbs AS, et al.** s.l. : Curr Opin Psychol, 2020;34:84-88.

24. *Insight into the relationship between sleep characteristics and anxiety: A cross-sectional study in indigenous and minority populations in northeastern Greece.* **Serdari A, et al.** s.l. : Psychiatry Res, 2020;292:113361.

25. *Anxiety and Depression in Patients with Obstructive Sleep Apnoea before and after Continuous Positive Airway Pressure: The ADIPOSA Study.* **Carneiro-Barrera A, et al.** s.l. : J Clin Med, 2019;8(12):2099.

26. *Obstructive Sleep Apnoea and Aortic Aneurysm: A Nationwide Population-Based Retrospective Study.* **Shih CC, et al.** s.l. : J Vasc Res, 2018;55(4):235-243.

27. *Prevalence of Obstructive Sleep Apnea in Patients with Thoracic Aortic Aneurysm: A Prospective, Parallel Cohort Study.* **Gaisl T, et al.** s.l. : Respiration, 2020;99(1):19-27.

28. *Asthma and Obstructive Sleep Apnea Overlap: What Has the Evidence Taught Us?* **Prasad B, et al.** s.l. : Am J Respir Crit Care Med, 2020;201(11):1345-1357.

29. *Association of obstructive sleep apnea with severity of patients hospitalized for acute asthma.* **Oka S, et al.** s.l. : Ann Allergy Asthma Immunol, 2020;124(2):165-170.e4.

30. *Asthma is associated with increased probability of needing CPAP in children with severe obstructive sleep apnea.* **Kilaikode S, et al.** s.l. : Pediatr Pulmonol, 2019;54(3):342-347.

31. *Prevalence, risk factors, and type of sleep apnea in patients with paroxysmal atrial fibrillation.* **Traaen, GM, et al.** s.l. : International journal of cardiology. Heart & vasculature, 2019, Vol. 26: 100447.

32. *CPAP is associated with decreased risk of AF recurrence in patients with OSA, especially those younger and slimmer: a meta-analysis.* **Yang Y, et al.** s.l. : J Interv Card Electrophysiol, 2020;58(3):369-379.

33. *Sleep-induced apnea syndrome. Prevalence of cardiac arrhythmias and their reversal after tracheostomy.* **Tilkian AG, et al.** s.l. : Am J Med, 1977;63(3):348-358.

34. *Association of high-risk scores for obstructive sleep apnea with symptomatic bradyarrhythmias.* **Velasco A, et al.** s.l. : J Cardiovasc Med (Hagerstown), 2014;15(5):407-410.

35. *Advanced atrioventricular block induced by obstructive sleep apnea before oxygen desaturation.* **Maeno K, et al.** s.l. : Heart Vessels, 2009;24(3):236-240.

36. *Symptoms of sleep disorders, inattention, and hyperactivity in children.* **Chervin RD, et al.** s.l. : Sleep, 1997;20(12):1185-1192.

37. *DSM-IV diagnoses and obstructive sleep apnea in children before and 1 year after adenotonsillectomy.* **Dillon JE, et al.** s.l. : Am Acad Child Adolesc Psychiatry, 2007;46(11):1425-1436.

38. ***Leggett CL, et alObstructive sleep apnea is a risk factor for Barrett's esophagus.*** *s.l. : Clin Gastroenterol Hepatol, 2014;12(4):583-8.e1.*

39. *Independent association of obstructive sleep apnea with Barrett's esophagus.* **Hadi YB, et al.** *s.l. : J Gastroenterol Hepatol, 2020;35(3):408-411.*

40. *The role of adenotonsillectomy in the treatment of primary nocturnal enuresis in children: A systematic review.* **Lehmann KJ, et al.** *s.l. : J Pediatr Urol, 2018;14(1):53.e1-53.e8.*

41. *Pre- and post-operative evaluation of the frequency of nocturnal enuresis and Modified Pediatric Epworth Scale in pediatric obstructive sleep apnea patients.* **Kaya KS, et al.** *s.l. : Int J Pediatr Otorhinolaryngol. , 2018;105:36-39.*

42. *Management and treatment of nocturnal enuresis-an updated standardization document from the International Children's Continence Society.* **Nevéus T, et al.** *s.l. : J Pediatr Urol, 2020;16(1):10-19.*

43. *Increased risk of benign prostate hyperplasia in sleep apnea patients: a nationwide population-based study.* **Chou PS, et al.** *s.l. : PLoS One, 2014 Mar 25;9(3):e93081.*

44. *Finasteride Use Is Associated with Higher Odds of Obstructive Sleep Apnea: Results from the US Food and Drug Administration Adverse Events Reporting System.* **al, Gupta MA et.** *s.l. : Skinmed, 2020 May 1;18(3):146-150.*

45. *Síndrome de apnea obstructiva del sueño en personas atendidas en consulta externa de psiquiatría: serie de casos [Obstructive sleep apnea syndrome in patients attending a psychiatry outpatient service: a case series].* **Tamayo Martínez N, Rosselli Cock D.** *s.l. : Rev Colomb Psiquiatr, 2017 Oct-Dec;46(4):243-246.*

46. *Clinical characteristics of obstructive sleep apnea in bipolar disorders.* **Geoffroy PA, et al.** *s.l. : J Affect Disord, 2019 Feb 15;245:1-7.*

47. *Risk of obstructive sleep apnea in patients with bipolar disorder: A nationwide population-based cohort study in Taiwan.* **Chang ET, et al.** *s.l. : 2019 Apr;73(4):163-168, Vol. Psychiatry Clin Neurosci.*

48. *Association between obstructive sleep apnoea and breast cancer: The Korean National Health Insurance Service Data 2007-2014.* **Choi JH, et al.** *s.l. : Sci Rep, 2019 Dec 13;9(1):19044.*

49. *Obstructive sleep apnea syndrome and causal relationship with female breast cancer: a mendelian randomization study.* **Gao XL, et al.** *s.l. : Aging (Albany NY), 2020 Feb 29;12(5):4082-4092.*

50. *ASSOCIATION OF OBSTRUCTIVE SLEEP APNEA WITH CENTRAL SEROUS CHORIORETINOPATHY AND CHOROIDAL THICKNESS: A Systematic Review and Meta-Analysis.* **Wu CY, et al.** *s.l. : Retina, 2018 Sep;38(9):1642-1651.*

51. *The Effect of Obstructive Sleep Apnea on Absolute Risk of Central Serous Chorioretinopathy.* **Pan CK, et al.** *s.l. : Am J Ophthalmol, 2020 Oct;218:148-155.*

52. *THE ASSOCIATION BETWEEN CENTRAL SEROUS CHORIORETINOPATHY AND SLEEP APNEA: A Nationwide Population-Based Study.* **Liu PK, et al.** *s.l. : Retina, 2020 Oct;40(10):2034-2044.*

53. *Associations Between Sleep Apnea and Subclinical Carotid Atherosclerosis: The Multi-Ethnic Study of Atherosclerosis. Stroke. 2019 Dec;50(12):3340-3346.* **al, Zhao YY et.**

54. *Prevalence of Sleep Apnea in Patients with Carotid Artery Stenosis.* **Nahorecki A, et al.** *s.l. : Adv Exp Med Biol, 2019;1211:69-75.*

55. *Association between the high risk for obstructive sleep apnea and intracranial carotid artery calcification in patients with acute ischemic stroke.* **Woo HG, et al.** *s.l. : Sleep Breath, 2020 Jun 19.*

56. *Effect of Heart Rate Variability on the Association Between the Apnea-Hypopnea Index and Cerebral Small Vessel Disease.* **Del Brutto OH, et al.** *s.l. : Stroke, 2019 Sep;50(9):2486-2491.*

57. *Subcortical ischaemic vascular dementia.* **Román GC, et al.** *s.l. : Lancet Neurol, 2002 Nov;1(7):426-36.*

58. *Genetic basis of sleep bruxism and sleep apnea-response to a medical puzzle.* **Wieckiewicz M, et al.** *s.l. : Sci Rep, 2020 May 4;10(1):7497.*

59. *Bruxism Relieved Under CPAP Treatment in a Patient With OSA Syndrome.* **Martinot JB, et al.** *s.l. : Chest, 2020 Mar;157(3):e59-e62.*

60. *The Relationship between Sleep Bruxism and Obstructive Sleep Apnea Based on Polysomnographic Findings.* **Martynowicz H, et al.** *s.l. : J Clin Med, 2019 Oct 11;8(10):1653.*

61. *Correlation between Parental-Reported Tooth Grinding and Sleep Disorders: Investigation in a Cohort of 741 Consecutive Children.* **Segù M, et al.** *s.l. : Pain Res Manag, 2020 Jul 30;2020:3408928.*

62. *Headache and sleep disorders: review and clinical implications for headache management.* **Rains JC, Poceta JS.** *s.l. : Headache, 2006 Oct;46(9):1344-63.*

63. *Improvement in cluster headache after treatment for obstructive sleep apnea.* **Zallek N, Chervin RD.** *s.l. : Sleep Med, 2000 Apr 1;1(2):135-138.*

64. *Clinical presentation, diagnosis and polysomnographic findings in children with migraine referred to sleep clinics.* **Domany KA, et al.** *s.l. : Sleep Med, 2019 Nov;63:57-63.*

65. *Predictors of chronic kidney disease in obstructive sleep apnea patients.* **Somkearti P, et al.** *s.l. : Multidiscip Respir Med, 2020 Jan 28;15(1):470.*

66. *Obstructive sleep apnea-hypopnea syndrome (OSAHS) comorbid with diabetes rather than OSAHS alone serves an independent risk factor for chronic kidney disease (CKD).* **Hui M, et al.** *s.l. : Ann Palliat Med, 2020 May;9(3):858-869.*

67. *Glomerular filtration rate in patients with obstructive sleep apnea: the influence of cystatin-C-based estimations and comorbidity.* **Nowiński A, et al.** *s.l. : J Thorac Dis, 2020 Mar;12(3):175-183.*

68. *Obstructive sleep apnea and Alzheimer's disease-related cerebrospinal fluid biomarkers in mild cognitive impairment.* **Díaz-Román M, et al.** *s.l. : Sleep, 2020 Jul 7;zsaa133.*

69. Obstructive sleep apnea, depression and cognitive impairment. **Vanek J, et al.** s.l. : Sleep Med, 2020 Mar 23;72:50-58.

70. Approach to the snoring child. **Tan YH, et al.** s.l. : Singapore Med J, 2020 Apr;61(4):170-175.

71. Oral Health and Oral Health-Related Quality of Life in Children With Obstructive Sleep Apnea. **Tamasas B, et al.** s.l. : J Clin Sleep Med, 2019 Mar 15;15(3):445-452.

72. Effects of obstructive sleep apnea and obesity on exercise function in children. **Evans CA, et al.** s.l. : Sleep, 2014; 37: 1103-1110.

73. Does obstructive sleep apnea affect exercise capacity and the hemodynamic response to exercise? An individual patient data and aggregate meta-analysis. **Berger M, et al.** s.l. : Sleep Med Rev. , 2019;45:42-53.

74. Nocturnal Hypoxemia is Associated With Low Testosterone Levels in Overweight Males and Older Men With Normal Weight. **Viana A, et al.** s.l. : J Clin Sleep Med, 2017 Dec 15;13(12):1395-1401.

75. Effect of 1 Week of Sleep Restriction on Testosterone Levels in Young Healthy Men. **Leproult R, van Cauter E.** s.l. : JAMA, 2011 Jun 1; 305(21): 2173–2174.

76. Association of Continuous Positive Airway Pressure Treatment With Sexual Quality of Life in Patients With Sleep Apnea: Follow-up Study of a Randomized Clinical Trial. **Jara SM, et al.** s.l. : JAMA Otolaryngol Head Neck Surg, 2018 Jul 1;144(7):587-593.

77. *Effects of nasal airway obstruction on facial growth.* **RM, Rubin.** *s.l. : Ear Nose Throat J, 1987 May;66(5):212-9.*

78. *Variation of patterns of malocclusion by site of pharyngeal obstruction in children.* **Nunes WR Jr, Di Francesco RC.** *s.l. : Arch Otolaryngol Head Neck Surg, 2010 Nov;136(11):1116-20.*

79. *Obstructive sleep apnea, depression and cognitive impairment.* **Vanek J, et al.** *s.l. : Sleep Med, 2020 Aug;72:50-58.*

80. *Continuous positive airway pressure can improve depression in patients with obstructive sleep apnoea syndrome: a meta-analysis based on randomized controlled trials.* **Yang X, et al.** *s.l. : J Int Med Res, 2020 Mar;48(3):300060519895096.*

81. *Anxiety and Depression in Patients with Obstructive Sleep Apnoea before and after Continuous Positive Airway Pressure: The ADIPOSA Study.* **Carneiro-Barrera A, et al.** *s.l. : J Clin Med, 2019 Dec 1;8(12):2099.*

82. *Obstructive sleep apnea is associated with depressive symptoms in pregnancy.* **Redhead K, et al.** *s.l. : Sleep, 2020 May 12;43(5):zsz270.*

83. *Obstructive Sleep Apnea Exacerbates Glucose Dysmetabolism and Pancreatic β-Cell Dysfunction in Overweight and Obese Nondiabetic Young Adults.* **Li N, et al.** *s.l. : Diabetes Metab Syndr Obes, 2020 Jul 10;13:2465-2476.*

84. Obstructive sleep apnea in patients with diabetes less than 40 years of age. **Soontornrungsun B, et al.** s.l. : Diabetes Metab Syndr, 2020 Sep 10;14(6):1859-1863.

85. Mortality and morbidity in obstructive sleep apnoea-hypopnoea syndrome: results from a 30-year prospective cohort study. **Dodds S, et al.** s.l. : ERJ Open Res, 2020 Sep 14;6(3):00057-2020.

86. Nocturnal oxygen desaturation in the late third trimester of uncomplicated pregnancy for prediction of late-onset gestational hypertension. **Watanabe M, et al.** s.l. : J Obstet Gynaecol Res, 2020 Jul 26.

87. Maternal Sleep-Disordered Breathing in Pregnancy and Increased Nocturnal Glucose Levels in Women with Gestational Diabetes. **Newbold R, et al.** s.l. : Chest, 2020 Jul 17;S0012-3692(20)31911-5.

88. Sleep Disorders are a Prevalent and Serious Comorbidity in Dry Eye. **Ayaki M, et al.** s.l. : Invest Ophthalmol Vis Sci, 2018;59(14):DES143-DES150.

89. Prevalence and risk factors of dry eye in 79,866 participants of the population-based Lifelines cohort study in the Netherlands. **Vehof J, et al.** s.l. : Ocul Surf, 2020;S1542-0124(20)30069-0.

90. Ocular surface assessment and morphological alterations in meibomian glands with meibography in obstructive sleep apnea Syndrome. **Karaca I, et al.** s.l. : Ocul Surf, 2019;17(4):771-776.

91. *Association between obstructive sleep apnea and atopic dermatitis in children: A nationwide, population-based cohort study.* **Hu JM, et al.** *s.l. : Pediatr Allergy Immunol, 2018;29(3):260-266.*

92. *Obstructive sleep apnea and the risk of atopic dermatitis: a population-based case control study. .* **Tien KJ, et al.** *s.l. : PLoS One, 2014;9(2):e89656.*

93. *Effect of obstructive sleep apnea hypopnea syndrome on lipid profile: a meta-regression analysis.* **Nadeem R, et al.** *s.l. : J Clin Sleep Med, 2014 May 15;10(5):475-89.*

94. *European Sleep Apnea Database collaborators. Long-term positive airway pressure therapy is associated with reduced total cholesterol levels in patients with obstructive sleep apnea: data from the European Sleep Apnea Database (ESADA).* **Gunduz C, et al.** *s.l. : Sleep Med, 2020 Mar 7;75:201-209.*

95. *Effect of Obstructive Sleep Apnea Treatment on Lipids in Obese Children.* **Amini Z, et al.** *s.l. : Children (Basel), 2017 Jun 1;4(6):44.*

96. *A critical analysis of the purported role of hypoxemia in the comorbidity of obstructive sleep apnea and epilepsy.* **Mishra P, et al.** *s.l. : Clin Physiol Funct Imaging, 2020 Oct 17.*

97. *Chronic intermittent hypoxia transiently increases hippocampal network activity in the gamma frequency band and 4-Aminopyridine-induced hyperexcitability in vitro.* **Villasana-Salazar B, et al.** *s.l. : Epilepsy Res, 2020 Oct;166:106375.*

98. *Vagus Nerve Stimulator (VNS)-induced Severe Obstructive Sleep Apnea Which Resolved After the VNS Was Turned Off.* **Gurung P, et al.** *s.l. : Cureus, 2020 Feb 6;12(2):e6901.*

99. *Urinary tract symptoms and erectile dysfunction in obstructive sleep apnea: Systematic review.* **Clerget A, et al.** *s.l. : Prog Urol, 2020 Aug 20:S1166-7087.*

100. *Effects of continuous positive airway pressure therapy on daytime and nighttime arterial blood pressure in patients with severe obstructive sleep apnea and endothelial dysfunction.* **Bischof F, et al.** *s.l. : Sleep Breath, 2020 Sep;24(3):941-951.*

101. *Continuous positive airway pressure therapy in obstructive sleep apnoea patients with erectile dysfunction-A meta-analysis.* **Yang Z, et al.** *s.l. : Clin Respir J, 2020 Sep 25.*

102. *Can continuous positive airway pressure improve lower urinary tract symptoms and erectile dysfunction in male patients with severe obstructive sleep apnea syndrome?* **Coban S.** *s.l. : Investig Clin Urol, 2020 Sep 24.*

103. *A new method for measuring daytime sleepiness: the Epworth sleepiness scale.* **MW, Johns.** *s.l. : Sleep, 1991 Dec;14(6):540-5.*

104. *Day-time drowsiness.* **JD, Parkes.** *s.l. : Lancet, 1981 Nov 28;2(8257):1213-8.*

105. *Is There a Link Between Obstructive Sleep Apnea Syndrome and Fibromyalgia Syndrome? .* **Köseoğlu Hİ, et al.** *s.l. : Turk Thorac J, 2017 Apr;18(2):40-46.*

106. Prevalence of obstructive sleep apnea in female patients with fibromyalgia. **Mutlu P, et al.** s.l. : Saudi Med J, 2020 Jul;41(7):740-745.

107. The relationship between floppy eyelid syndrome and obstructive sleep apnoea. **Muniesa MJ, et al.** s.l. : Br J Ophthalmol, 2013 Nov;97(11):1387-90.

108. Prospective Evaluation of Floppy Eyelid Syndrome at Baseline and after CPAP Therapy. **Vieira MJ, et al.** s.l. : Curr Eye Res, 2020 Jun 16;1-4.

109. Links between obstructive sleep apnea and glaucoma neurodegeneration. **Cesareo M, et al.** s.l. : Prog Brain Res, 2020;257:19-36.

110. Obstructive sleep apnea as a risk factor for primary open angle glaucoma and ocular hypertension in a monocentric pilot study. **Bahr K, et al.** s.l. : Respir Res, 2020 Oct 8;21(1):258.

111. Long-term Effect of Continuous Positive Air Pressure Therapy on Intraocular Pressure in Patients with Primary Open-angle Glaucoma with Obstructive Sleep Apnea. **Hirunpatravong P, et al.** s.l. : J Curr Glaucoma Pract, 2019 Sep-Dec;13(3):94-98.

112. Obstructive sleep apnea syndrome and growth failure. **Esteller E, et al.** s.l. : Int J Pediatr Otorhinolaryngol, 2018 May;108:214-218.

113. The effect of adenotonsillectomy on serum insulin like growth factors and the adenoid/nasopharynx ratio in pediatric patients: a blind, prospective clinical study.

Tatlıpınar A, et al. *s.l.* : *Int J Pediatr Otorhinolaryngol, 2012 Feb;76(2):248-52.*

114. Changes in serum IGF-1 and IGFBP-3 levels and growth in children following adenoidectomy, tonsillectomy or adenotonsillectomy. **Kiris M, et al.** *s.l.* : *2010 May;74(5):528-31, Vol. Int J Pediatr Otorhinolaryngol.*

115. Intermittent Hypoxia and Hypercapnia, a Hallmark of Obstructive Sleep Apnea, Alters the Gut Microbiome and Metabolome. **Tripathi A, et al.** *s.l.* : *mSystems, 2018 Jun 5;3(3):e00020.*

116. Gut microbiota in obstructive sleep apnea-hypopnea syndrome: disease-related dysbiosis and metabolic comorbidities. **Ko CY, et al.** *s.l.* : *Clin Sci (Lond), 2019 Apr 12;133(7):905-917.*

117. Obstructive Sleep Apnea and Systemic Hypertension: Gut Dysbiosis as the Mediator? . **Mashaqi S, Gozal D.** *s.l.* : *J Clin Sleep Med, 2019 Oct 15;15(10):1517-1527.*

118. Bugs, breathing and blood pressure: microbiota-gut-brain axis signalling in cardiorespiratory control in health and disease. **O'Connor KM, et al.** *s.l.* : *J Physiol, 2020 Jul 11. doi: 10.1113/JP280279.*

119. The effect of intermittent hypoxia and fecal microbiota of OSAS on genes associated with colorectal cancer. **Gao J, et al.** *s.l.* : *Sleep Breath, 2020 Oct 7. doi: 10.1007/s11325-020-02204-z.*

120. *Increased eustachian tube dysfunction in infants with obstructive sleep apnea.* **Robison JG, et al.** *s.l. : Laryngoscope, 2012 May;122(5):1170-7.*

121. *he association between obstructive sleep apnea and hearing loss: a cross-sectional analysis.* **Kayabasi S, et al.** *s.l. : Eur Arch Otorhinolaryngol, 2019 Aug;276(8):2215-2221.*

122. *Inner ear function in patients with obstructive sleep apnea.* **Li X, et al.** *s.l. : Sleep Breath, 2020 Mar;24(1):65-69.*

123. *Evaluation of the changes in the hearing system over the years among patients with OSAS using a CPAP device.* **Deniz M, Ersözlü T.** *s.l. : Cranio, 2020 Jun 28:1-4.*

124. *Clinical and polysomnographic features of hypertension in obstructive sleep apnea: A single-center cross-sectional study.* **Gürün Kaya A, et al.** *s.l. : Anatol J Cardiol, 2020 Jun;23(6):334-341.*

125. *Sleep Apnea, Hypertension and the Sympathetic Nervous System in the Adult Population.* **Venkataraman S, et al.** *s.l. : J Clin Med, 2020 Feb 21;9(2):591.*

126. *Incidence of hypertension in obstructive sleep apnea using hypopneas defined by 3 percent oxygen desaturation or arousal but not by only 4 percent oxygen desaturation.* **Budhiraja R, et al.** *s.l. : J Clin Sleep Med, 2020 Oct 15;16(10):1753-1760.*

127. *Impact of CPAP on arterial stiffness in patients with obstructive sleep apnea: a meta-analysis of randomized trials.* **Chalegre ST, et al.** *s.l. : Sleep Breath, 2020 Oct 22. doi: 10.1007/s11325-020-02226-7.*

128. *Effect of Sleep Disorders on Blood Pressure and Hypertension in Children.* **DelRosso LM, et al.** *s.l. : Curr Hypertens Rep, 2020 Sep 7;22(11):88.*

129. *Childhood OSA is an independent determinant of blood pressure in adulthood: longitudinal follow-up study.* **Chan KC, et al.** *s.l. : Thorax, 2020 May;75(5):422-431.*

130. *Association Between Hypercoagulability and Severe Obstructive Sleep Apnea.* **Hong SN, et al.** *s.l. : JAMA Otolaryngol, Head Neck Surg. 2017 Oct 1;143(10):996-1002.*

131. *Sleep apnea and venous thromboembolism. A systematic review.* **Lippi G, et al.** *s.l. : Thromb Haemost, 2015 Nov;114(5):958-63.*

132. *Three-year changes of prothrombotic factors in a cohort of South Africans with a high clinical suspicion of obstructive sleep apnea.* **von Känel R, et al.** *s.l. : Thromb Haemost, 2016 Jan;115(1):63-72.*

133. *The Plasminogen System and Transforming Growth Factor-ß in Subjects With Obstructive Sleep Apnea Syndrome: Effects of CPAP Treatment.* **Steffanina A, et al.** *s.l. : Respir Care, 2015 Nov;60(11):1643-51.*

134. *Prevalence of newly established thyroid disorders in patients with moderate-to-severe obstructive sleep apnea syndrome.* **Bruyneel M, et al.** *s.l. : Sleep Breath, 2019 Jun;23(2):567-573.*

135. *Hypothyroidism and Its Association With Sleep Apnea Among Adults in the United States: NHANES 2007-2008.*

Thavaraputta S, et al. s.l. : J Clin Endocrinol Metab, 2019 Nov 1;104(11):4990-4997.

*136. Association of Irritable Bowel Syndrome and Sleep Apnea in Patients Referred to Sleep Laboratory. **Ghiasi F, et al.** s.l. : J Res Med Sci, 2017 Jun 21;22:72.*

*137. Polysomnographic and Actigraphic Evidence of Sleep Fragmentation in Patients With Irritable Bowel Syndrome. **Rotem AY, et.** s.l. : Sleep, 2003 Sep;26(6):747-52.*

*138. Medical Literature Implies Continuous Positive Airway Pressure Might Be Appropriate Treatment for Irritable Bowel Syndrome. **Herr, JR.** s.l. : Chest, 2002 Sep;122(3):1107.*

*139. CPAP treats muscle cramps in patients with obstructive sleep apnea. **Westwood AJ, et al.** s.l. : J Clin Sleep Med, 2014 Jun 15;10(6):691-2.*

*140. Obstructive Sleep Apnea and Testosterone Deficiency. **Kim SD, et al.** s.l. : World J Mens Health, 2019 Jan;37(1):12-18.*

*141. Obstructive sleep apnea is not an independent determinant of testosterone in men. **Clarke BM, et al.** s.l. : Eur J Endocrinol, 2020 Jul;183(1):31-39.*

*142. Effects of CPAP on Testosterone Levels in Patients With Obstructive Sleep Apnea: A Meta-Analysis Study. **Cignarelli A, et al.** s.l. : Front Endocrinol (Lausanne), 2019 Aug 21;10:551.*

*143. Sleep Apnea and Cancer: Analysis of a Nationwide Population Sample. **Gozal D, et al.** s.l. : Sleep, 2016 Aug 1;39(8):1493-500.*

144. Biomarkers of carcinogenesis and tumour growth in patients with cutaneous melanoma and obstructive sleep apnoea. **Santamaria-Martos F, et al.** s.l. : Eur Respir J, 2018 Mar 15;51(3):1701885.

145. Intermittent hypoxia promotes melanoma lung metastasis via oxidative stress and inflammation responses in a mouse model of obstructive sleep apnea. **Li L, et al.** s.l. : Respir Res, 2018 Feb 12;19(1):28.

146. Soluble PD-L1 is a potential biomarker of cutaneous melanoma aggressiveness and metastasis in obstructive sleep apnoea patients. **Cubillos-Zapata C, et al.** s.l. : Eur Respir J, 2019 Jan 31;53(2):1801298.

147. Sleep-Disordered Breathing in People with Multiple Sclerosis: Prevalence, Pathophysiological Mechanisms, and Disease Consequences. **Hensen HA, et al.** s.l. : Front Neurol, 2018 Jan 15;8:740.

148. Association between obstructive sleep apnea syndrome and nocturia: a meta-analysis. **Zhou J, et al.** s.l. : Sleep Breath, 2020 Jan 6. doi: 10.1007/s11325-019-01981-6.

149. Obstructive Sleep Apnea Syndrome as a Potential Cause of Nocturia in Younger Adults. **Miyauchi Y, et al.** s.l. : Urology, 2020 Sep;143:42-47.

150. Prevalence of Screening High Risk of Obstructive Sleep Apnea Among Urogynecology Patients. **Myer ENB, et al.** s.l. : Female Pelvic Med Reconstr Surg, 2020 Aug;26(8):503-507.

151. The effect of continuous positive airway pressure on nocturia in patients with obstructive sleep apnea syndrome.

Vrooman OPJ, et al. s.l. : Neurourol Urodyn, 2020 Apr;39(4):1124-1128.

152. Association between non-alcoholic fatty liver disease and obstructive sleep apnea. **Umbro I, et al.** s.l. : World J Gastroenterol, 2020 May 28;26(20):2669-2681.

153. Association between obstructive sleep apnea and non-alcoholic fatty liver disease in pediatric patients: a meta-analysis. **Chen LD, et al.** s.l. : Pediatr Obes, 2020 Sep 2:e12718.

154. CPAP Did Not Improve Nonalcoholic Fatty Liver Disease in Patients with Obstructive Sleep Apnea: A Randomized Clinical Trial. **Ng SS, et al.** s.l. : Am J Respir Crit Care Med, 2020 Sep 14. doi: 10.1164/rccm.202005-1868OC.

155. Obstructive sleep apnoea and increased risk of non-arteritic anterior ischaemic optic neuropathy. **Yang HK, et al.** s.l. : Br J Ophthalmol, 2019 Aug;103(8):1123-1128.

156. Nonarteritic anterior ischaemic optic neuropathy and its association with obstructive sleep apnoea: a health insurance database study. **Sun MH, et al.** s.l. : Acta Ophthalmol, 2019 Feb;97(1):e64-e70.

157. Structural assessment of the optic nerve in patients with obstructive sleep apnea syndrome: Case-control study. **Uslu H, et al.** s.l. : Eur J Ophthalmol, 2020 Jun 2:1120672120926859.

158. Overactive bladder in women with sleep apnoea-hipopnea syndrome. **Grau N, et al.** s.l. : European Respiratory Journal, 2012 40: P1894.

159. *Effect of Continuous Positive Airway Pressure on Overactive Bladder Symptoms in Patients with Obstructive Sleep Apnea Syndrome.* **Dinç ME, et al.** s.l. : Turk Arch Otorhinolaryngol, 2018;56(3):133-138.

160. *Parkinson's disease: A systematic review and meta-analysis of polysomnographic findings.* **Zhang Y, et al.** s.l. : Sleep Med Rev , 2020;51:101281.

161. *Obstructive sleep apnea in Parkinson's disease: a study in 239 Chinese patients.* **Shen Y, et al.** s.l. : Sleep Med, 2020;67:237-243.

162. *Neurodegenerative Disorders: Current Evidence in Support of Benefit from Sleep Apnea Treatment.* **Lajoie AC, et al.** s.l. : J Clin Med, 2020;9(2):297.

163. *Association Between Periodontal Disease and Obstructive Sleep Apnea: What the Periodontist Should Know.* **Price R, Kang P.** s.l. : Compend Contin Educ Dent, 2020;41(3):149-154.

164. *Risk of developing obstructive sleep apnea among women with polycystic ovarian syndrome: a nationwide longitudinal follow-up study.* **Lin TY, e al.** s.l. : Sleep Med, 2017 Aug;36:165-169.

165. *The prevalence of obstructive sleep apnoea in women with polycystic ovary syndrome: a systematic review and meta-analysis.* **Kahal H, et al.** s.l. : Sleep Breath, 2020 Mar;24(1):339-350.

166. *The relationship between obstructive sleep apnoea and quality of life in women with polycystic ovary syndrome: a*

cross-sectional study. **Kahal H, et al.** s.l. : Ther Adv Endocrinol Metab, 2020 Feb 21;11:2042018820906689.

167. Sleep Disorders in Early Psychosis: Incidence, Severity, and Association With Clinical Symptoms. **Reeve S, et al.** s.l. : Schizophr Bull, 2019 Mar 7;45(2):287-295.

168. Sleep disturbance: a potential target to improve symptoms and quality of life in those living with psychosis. **Boland C, et al.** s.l. : Ir J Psychol Med, 2020 Jan 14:1-6.

169. Risk of obstructive sleep apnea in patients with schizophrenia: a nationwide population-based cohort study. **Wu YY, et al.** s.l. : Soc Psychiatry Psychiatr Epidemiol, 2020 Dec;55(12):1671-1677.

170. Cognition in schizophrenia improves with treatment of severe obstructive sleep apnoea: A pilot study. **Myles H, et al.** s.l. : Schizophr Res Cogn, 2018 Nov 6;15:14-20.

171. Obstructive sleep apnea and the risk of autoimmune diseases: a longitudinal population-based study. **Kang JH, et al.** s.l. : Sleep Med, 2012 Jun;13(6):583-8.

172. The complex associations between obstructive sleep apnea and auto-immune disorders: A review. **Vakil M, et al.** s.l. : Med Hypotheses, 2018 Jan;110:138-143.

173. Airways therapy of obstructive sleep apnea dramatically improves aberrant levels of soluble cytokines involved in autoimmune disease. **Phillips BG, et al.** s.l. : Clin Immunol, 2020 Oct 2;221:108601.

174. Impact of adenotonsillectomy on the dentofacial development of obstructed children: a systematic review and meta-analysis. **Becking BE, et al.** s.l. : Eur J Orthod, 2017 Oct 1;39(5):509-518.

Made in United States
Orlando, FL
26 July 2024

49569518R00085